Welcome to "Serenity Circles," a captivating mandala coloring book designed for adults and teens seeking tranquility, creativity, and inner balance. Dive into the mesmerizing world of mandalas, where each intricate pattern invites you to explore mindfulness, self-expression, and relaxation.

Benefits of "Serenity Circles":

1. **Stress Relief and Anxiety Reduction:** As you immerse yourself in coloring these harmonious designs, your mind gently unwinds. The rhythmic motion of filling in the circles soothes your soul, easing tension and promoting calmness.
2. **Mindful Meditation:** Mandalas have been used for centuries as tools for meditation. By focusing on the symmetrical shapes and intricate details, you enter a state of mindfulness—a respite from the chaos of daily life.
3. **Increased Self-Awareness:** Each layer of a mandala represents a different aspect of life. As you color, reflect on your own journey—your joys, challenges, and aspirations. Discover hidden insights and connect with your inner self.
4. **Boosted Creativity:** The circular patterns encourage your imagination to flow freely. Experiment with colors, shading, and blending techniques. There are no rules—just pure creative expression.
5. **Art Therapy:** "Serenity Circles" is more than a coloring book; it's a therapeutic experience. Engage your senses, feel the texture of the paper, and let the colors transport you to a serene realm.
6. **Self-Confidence:** Coloring outside the lines? Embrace it! Mandala celebrate imperfection. Trust your instincts, and let your intuition guide your choices. Your unique interpretation is a masterpiece in itself.
7. **Stabilized Blood Pressure:** Studies suggest that coloring mandalas can help regulate blood pressure. <u>The gentle focus required during coloring promotes relaxation and overall well-being</u> (1).

(**1**): **The surprising mandala coloring benefits for adults - happiness.com**

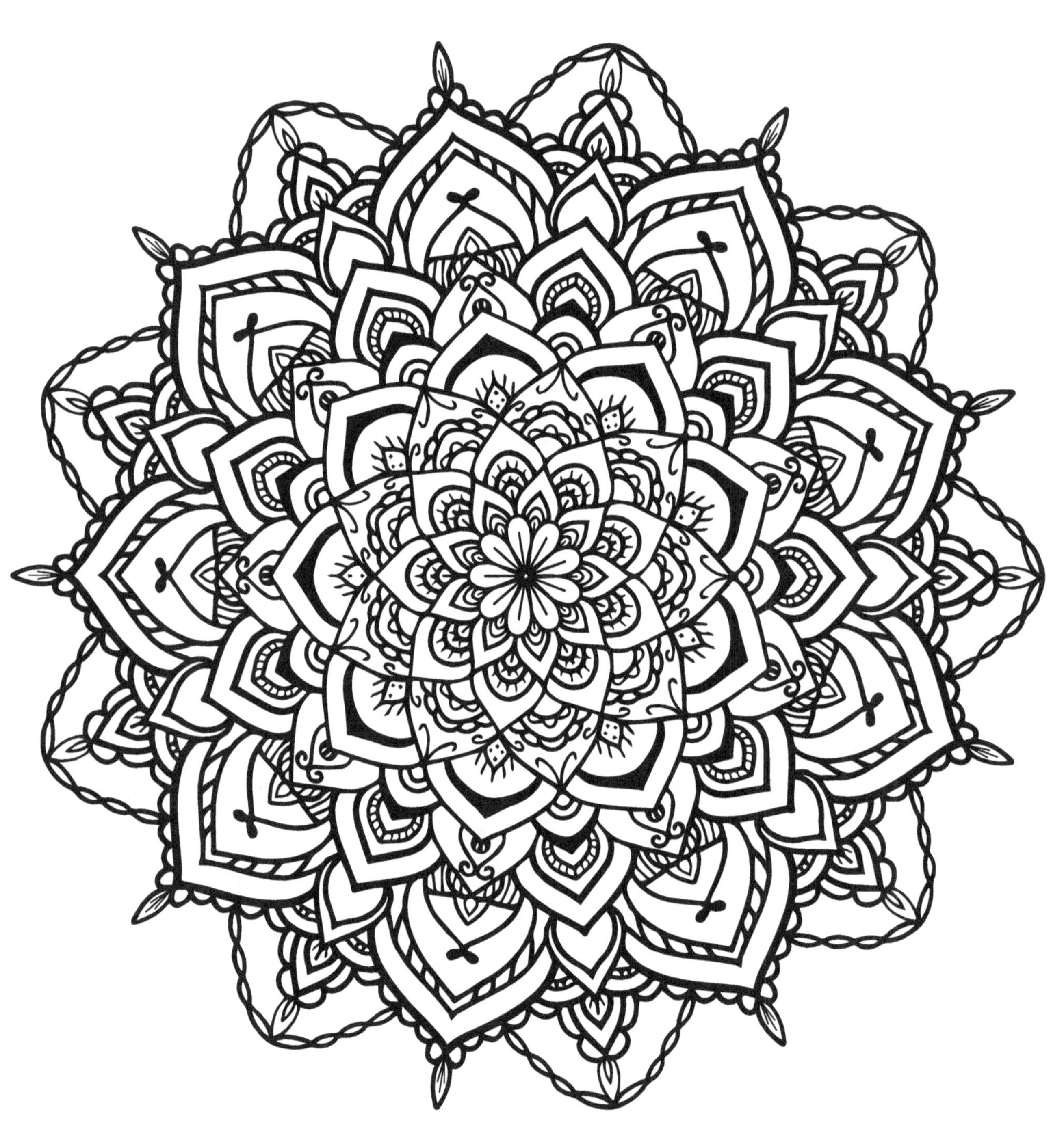

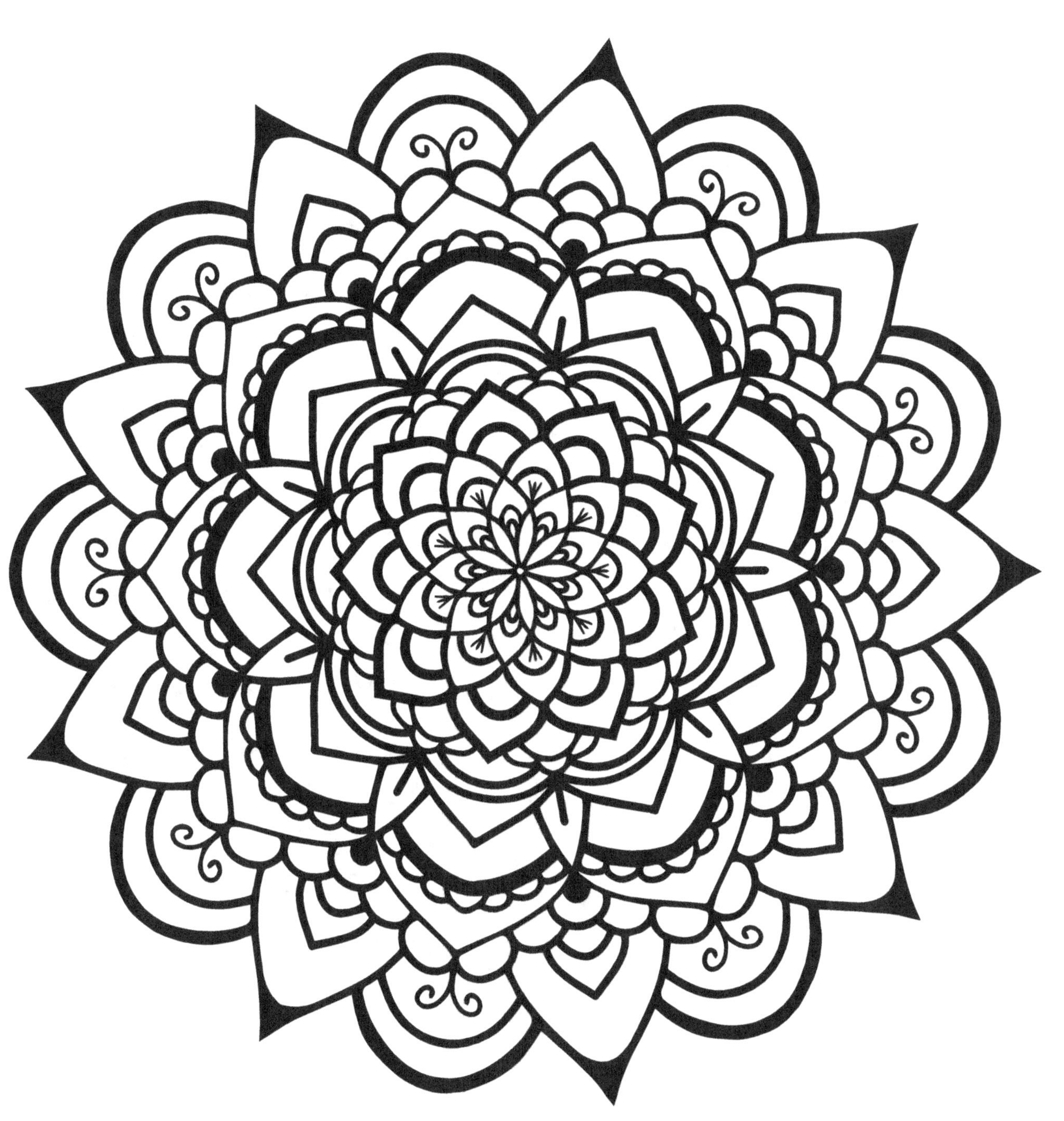

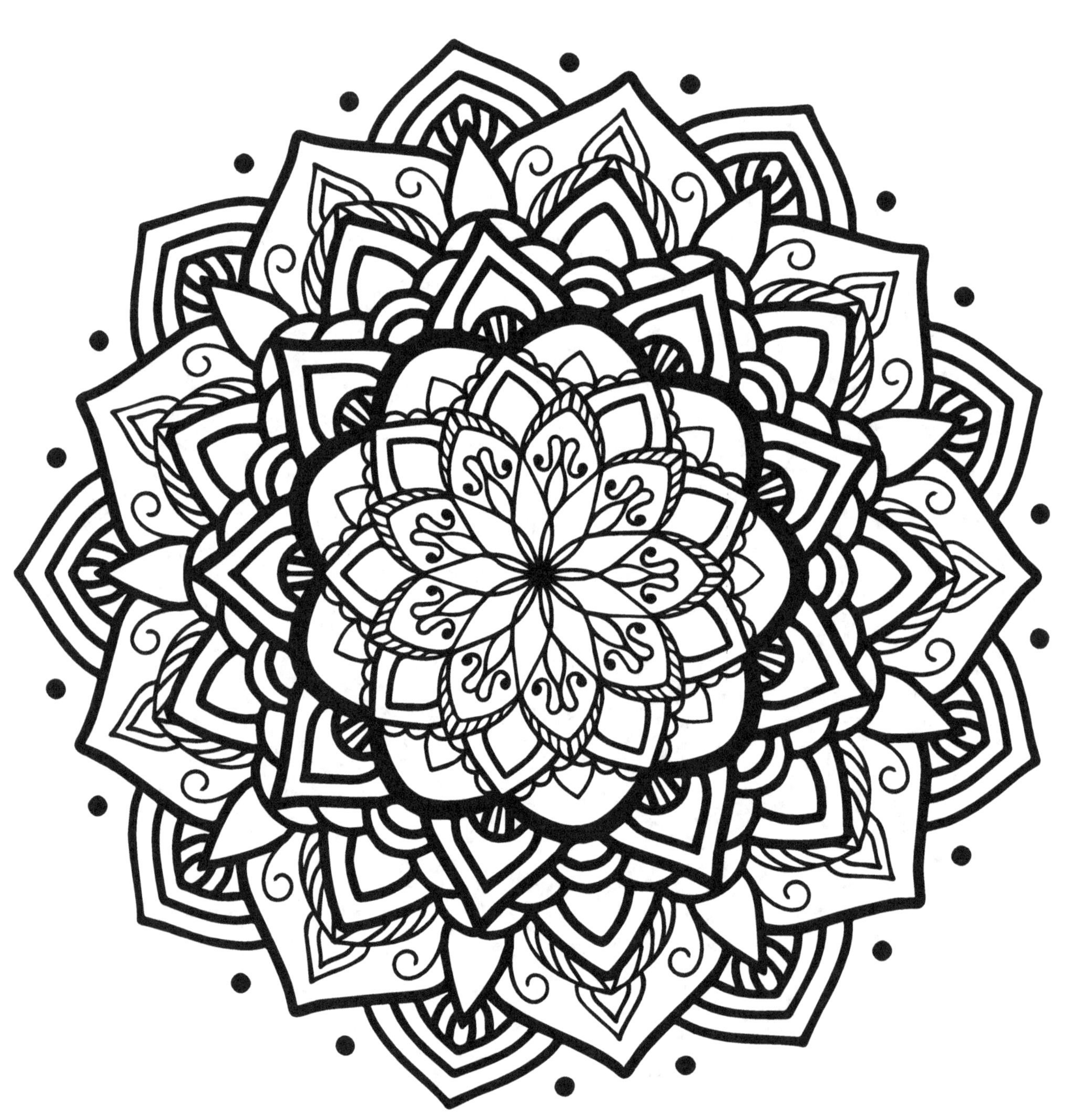

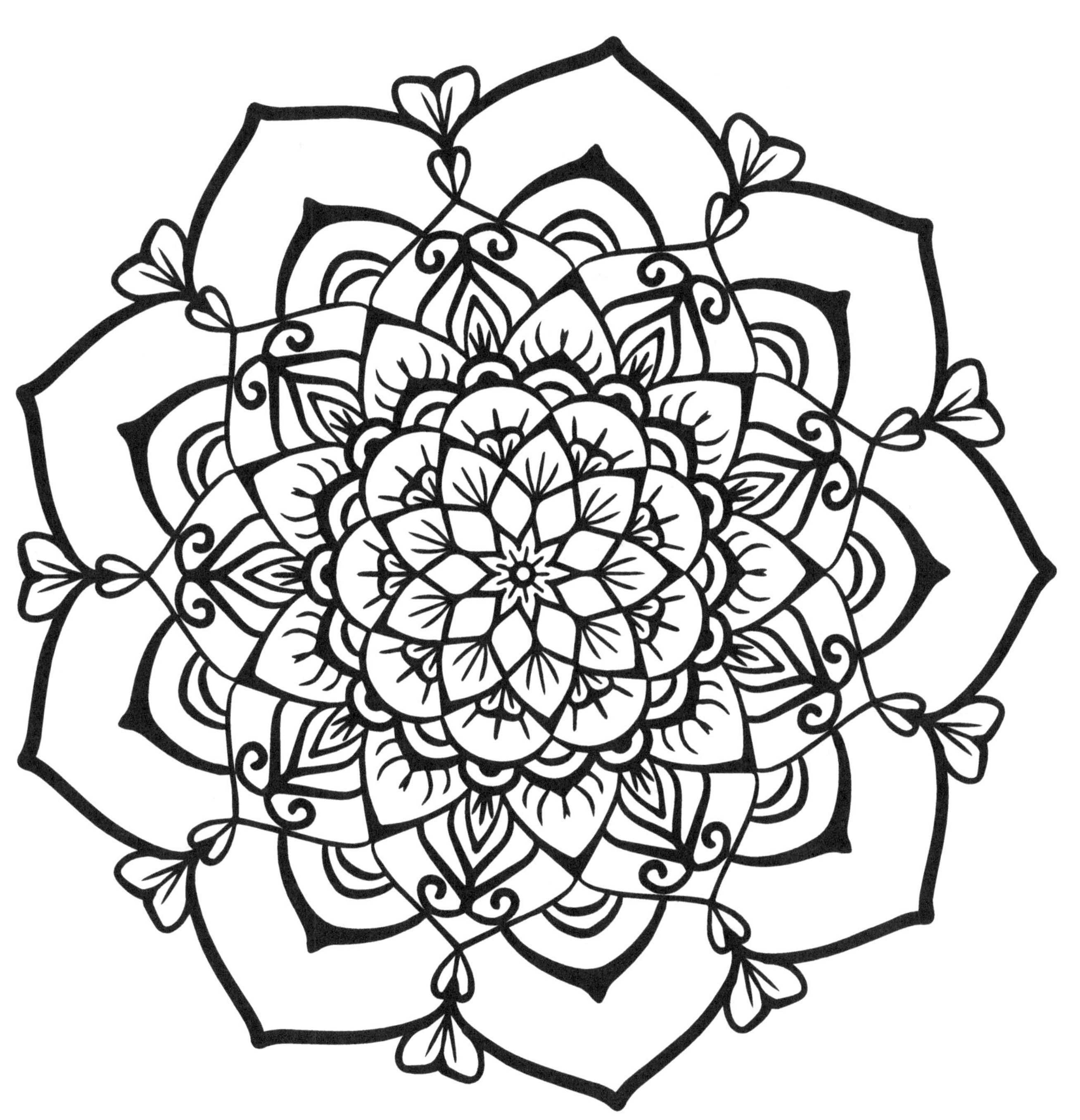

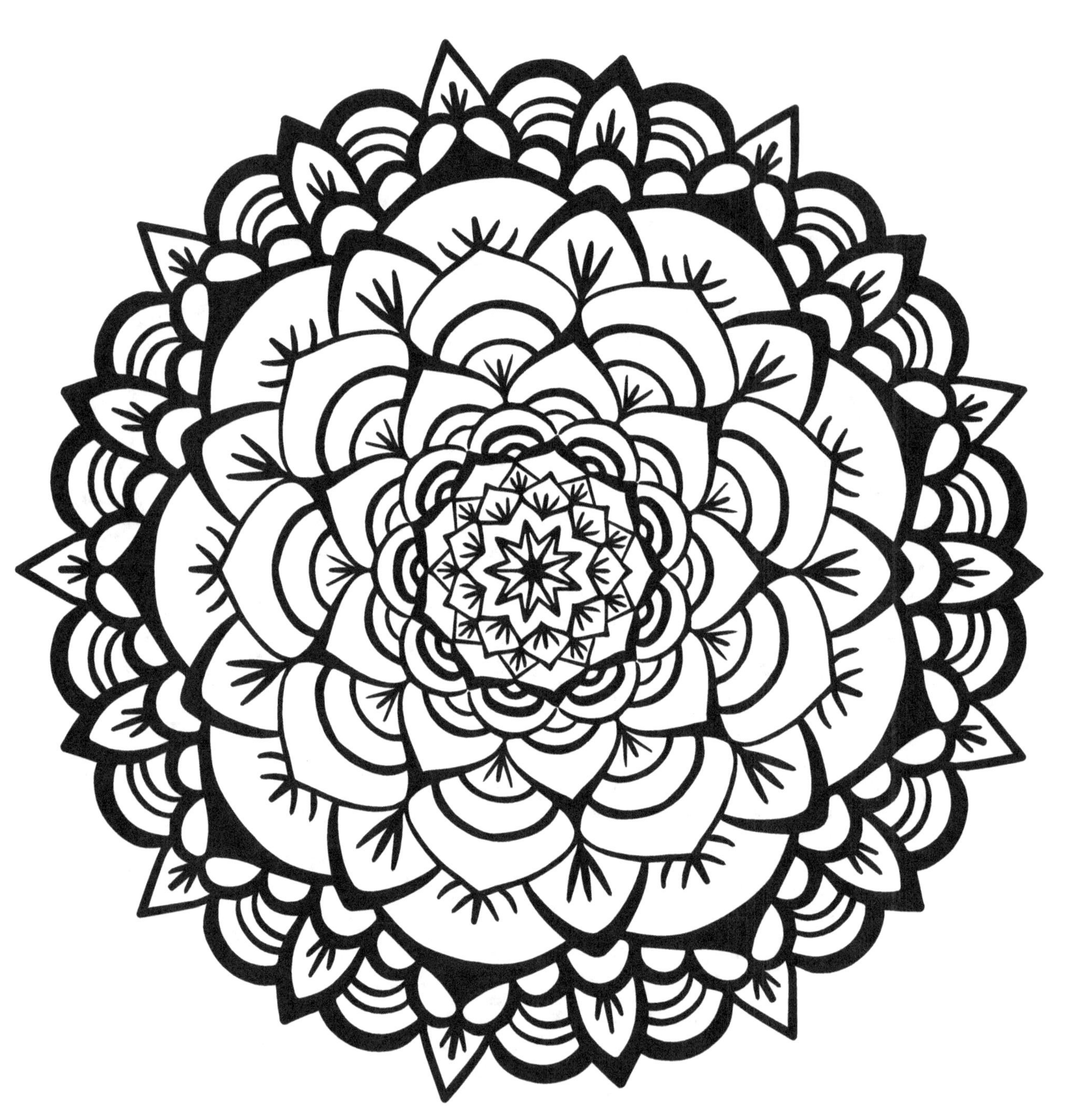

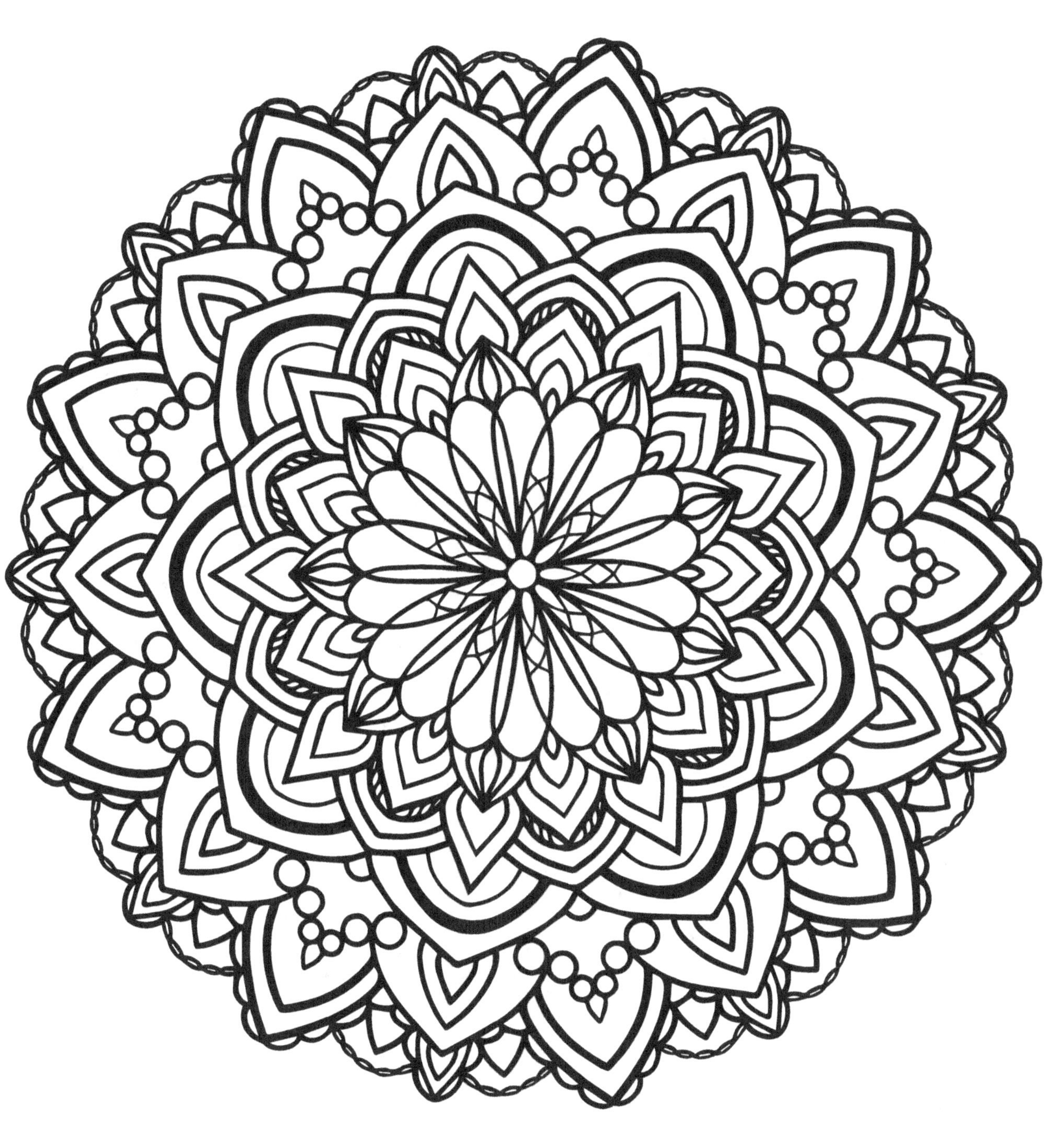

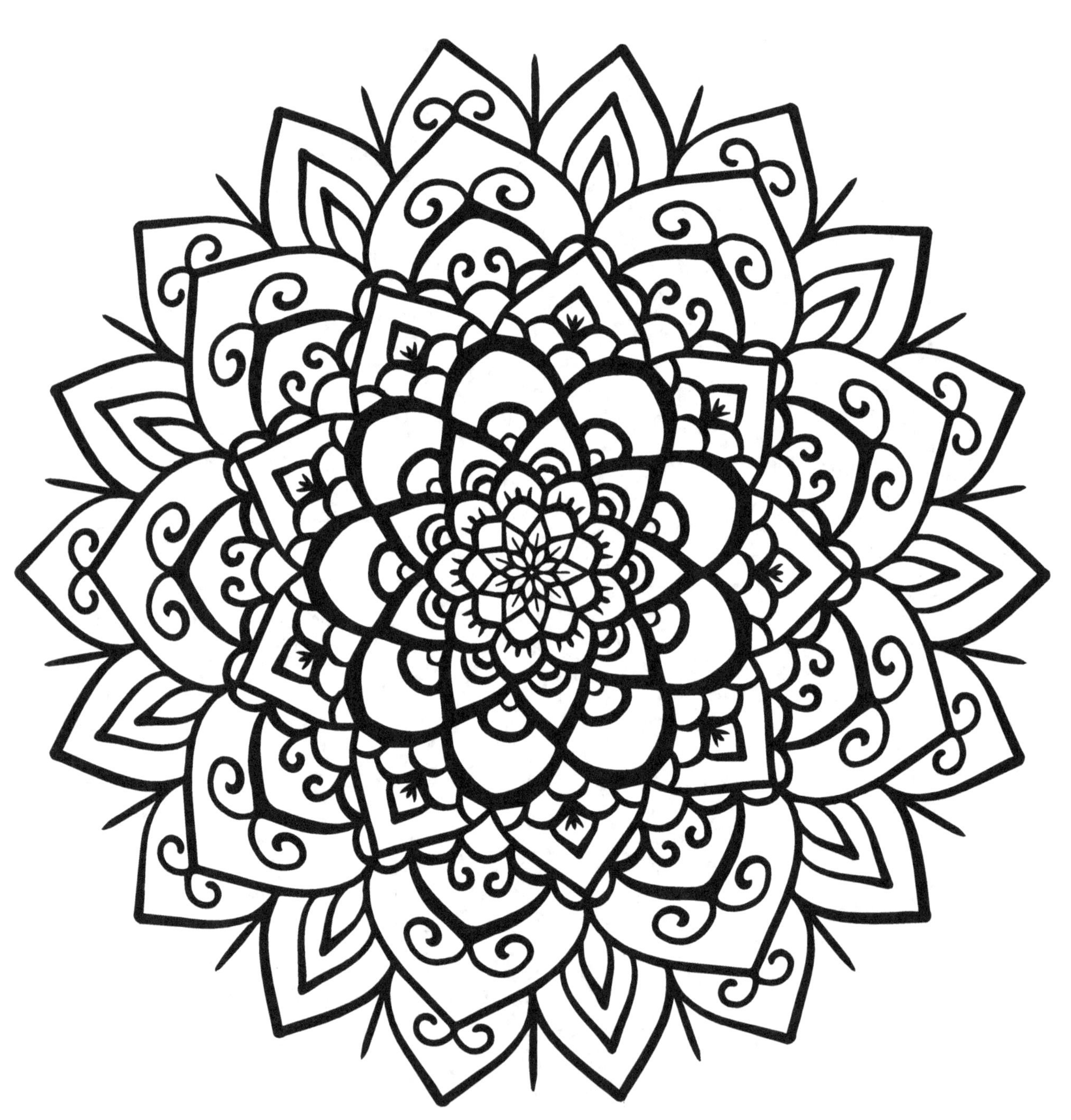

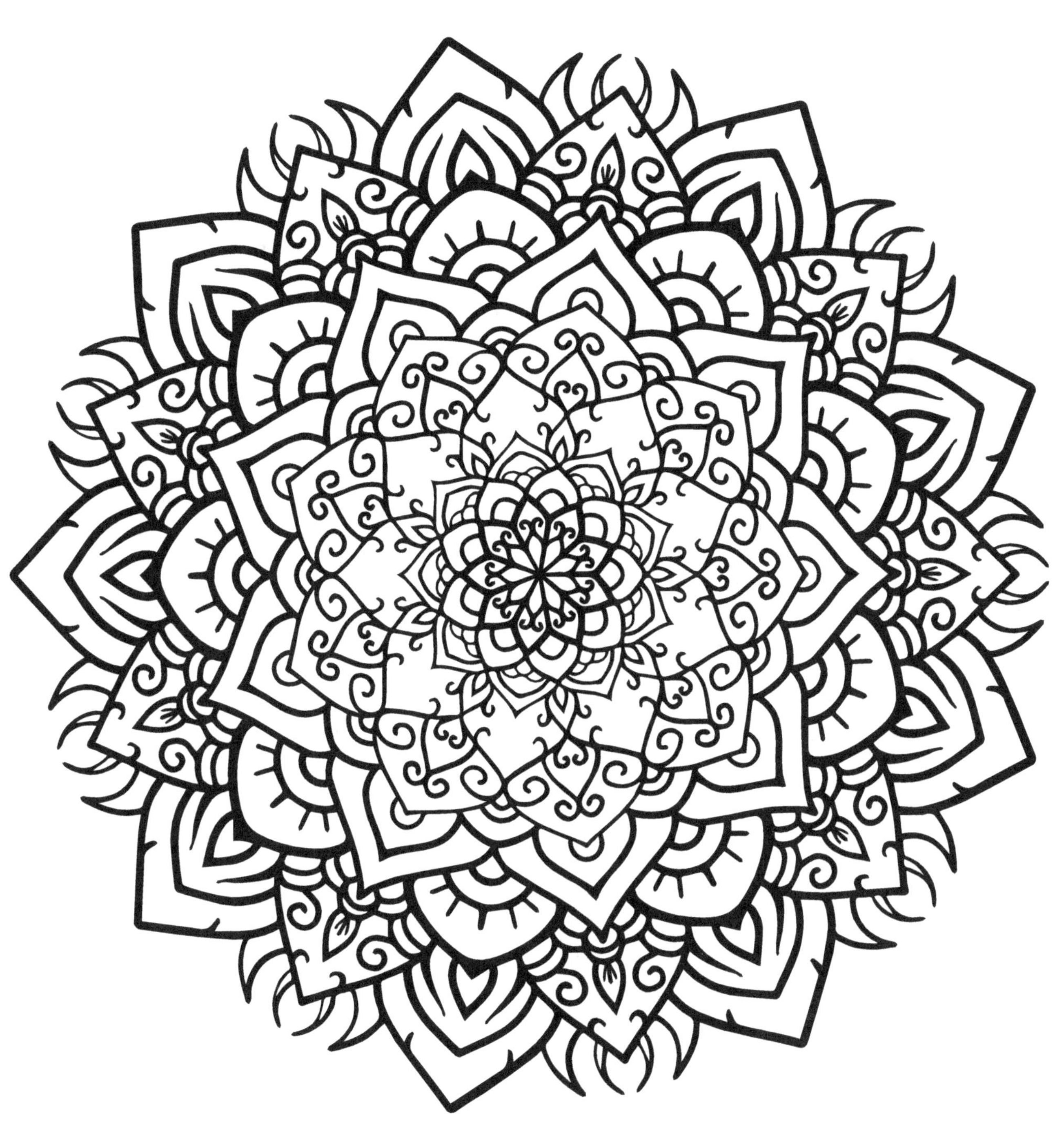

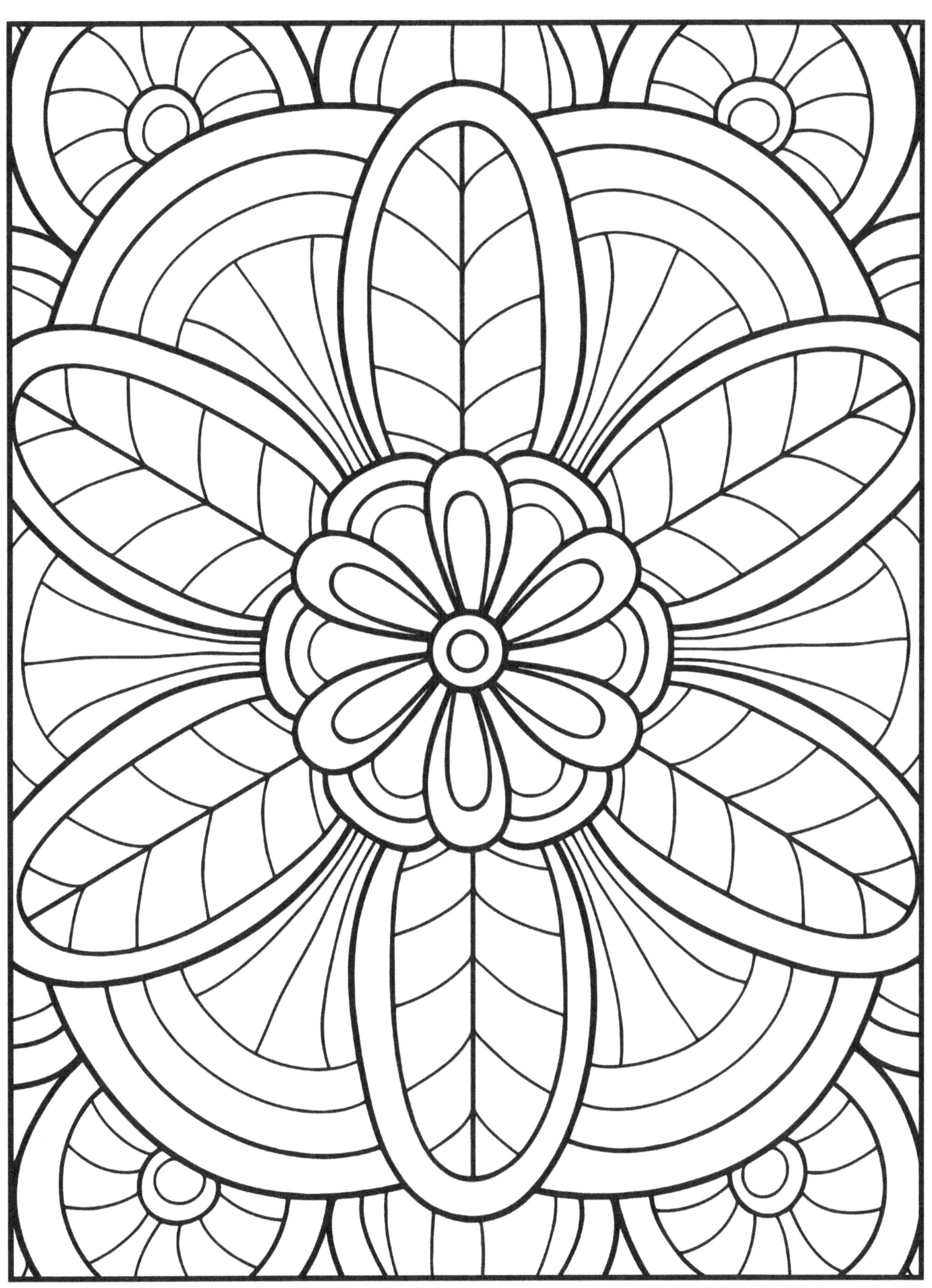

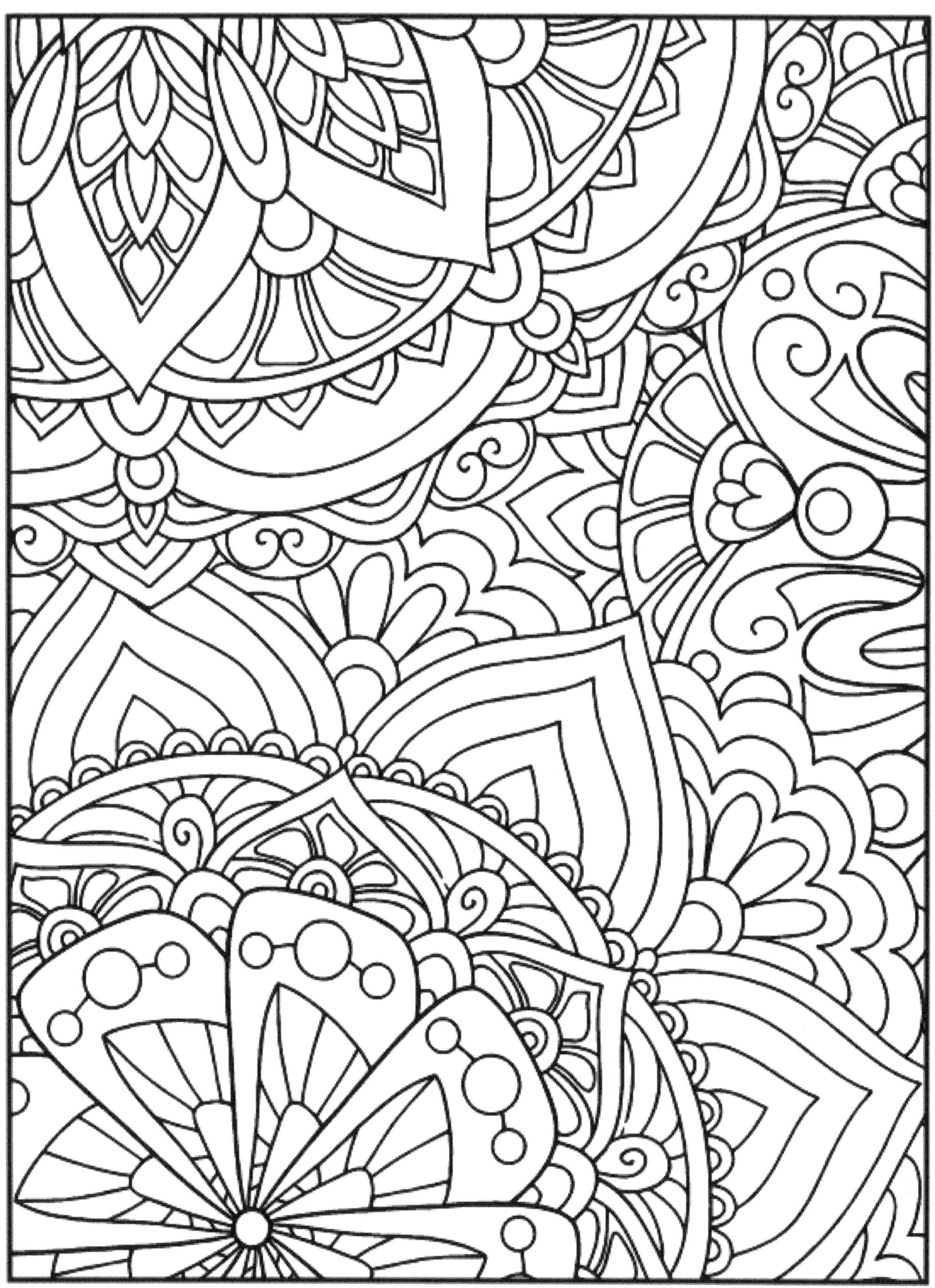

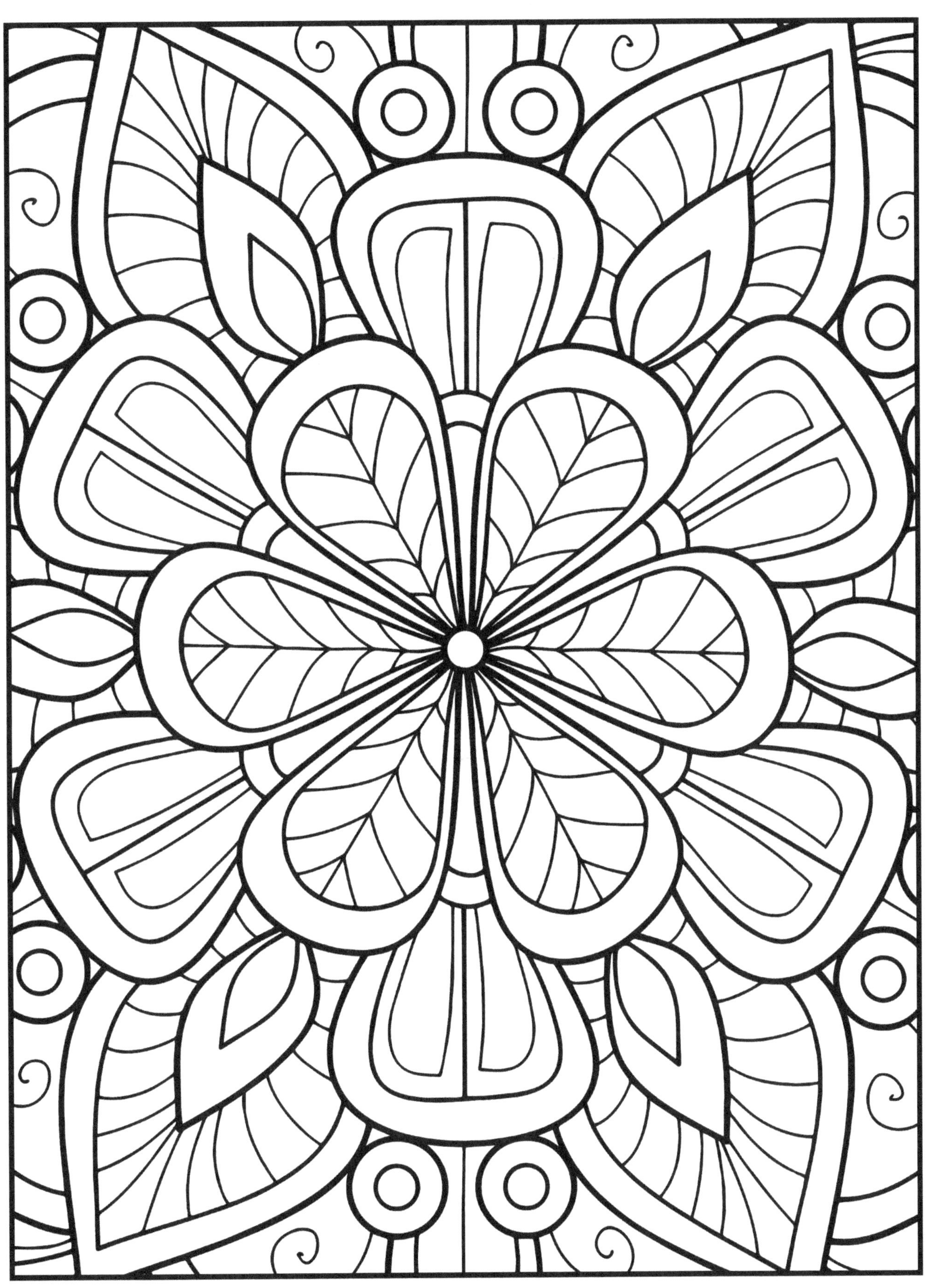

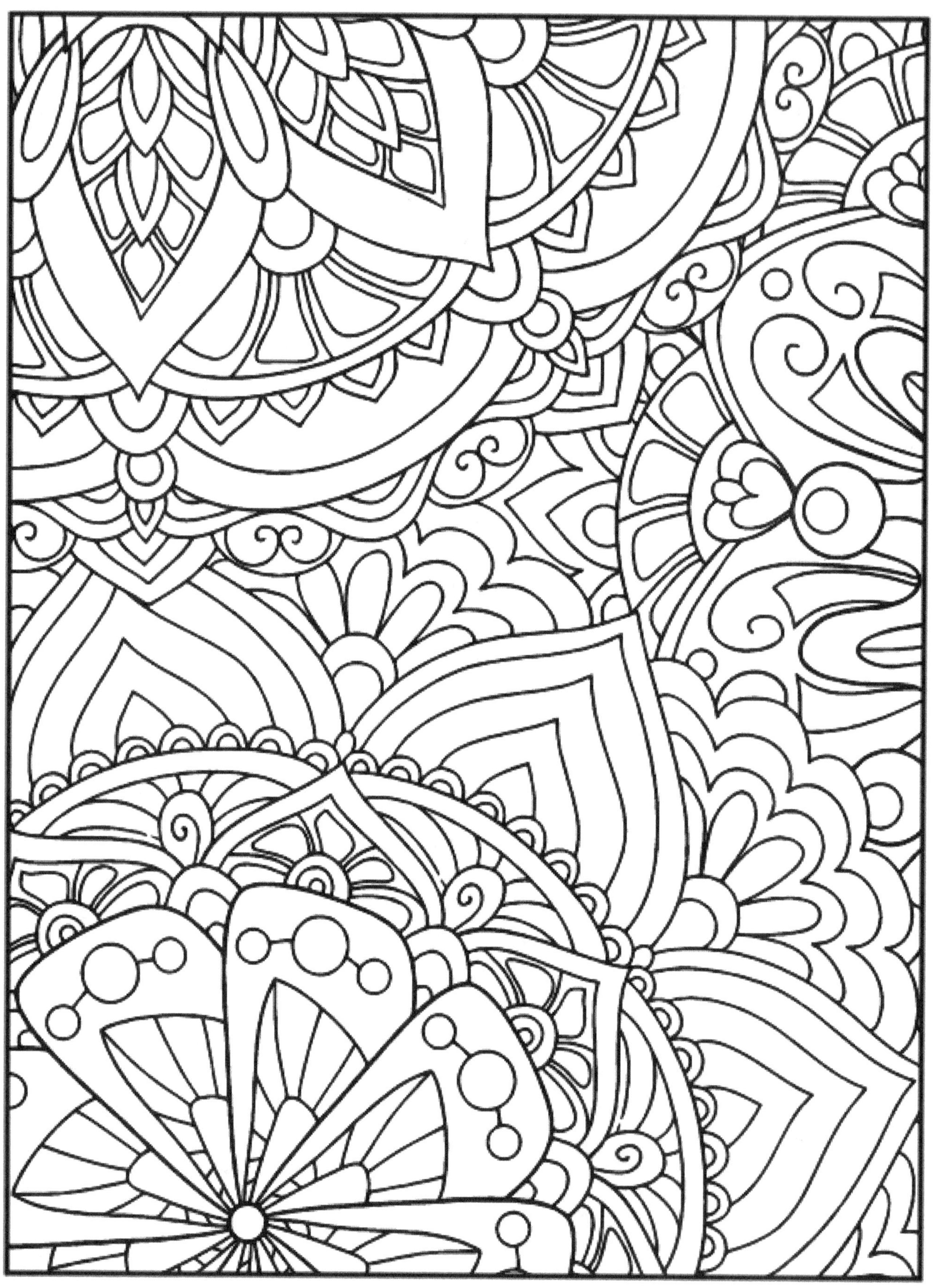

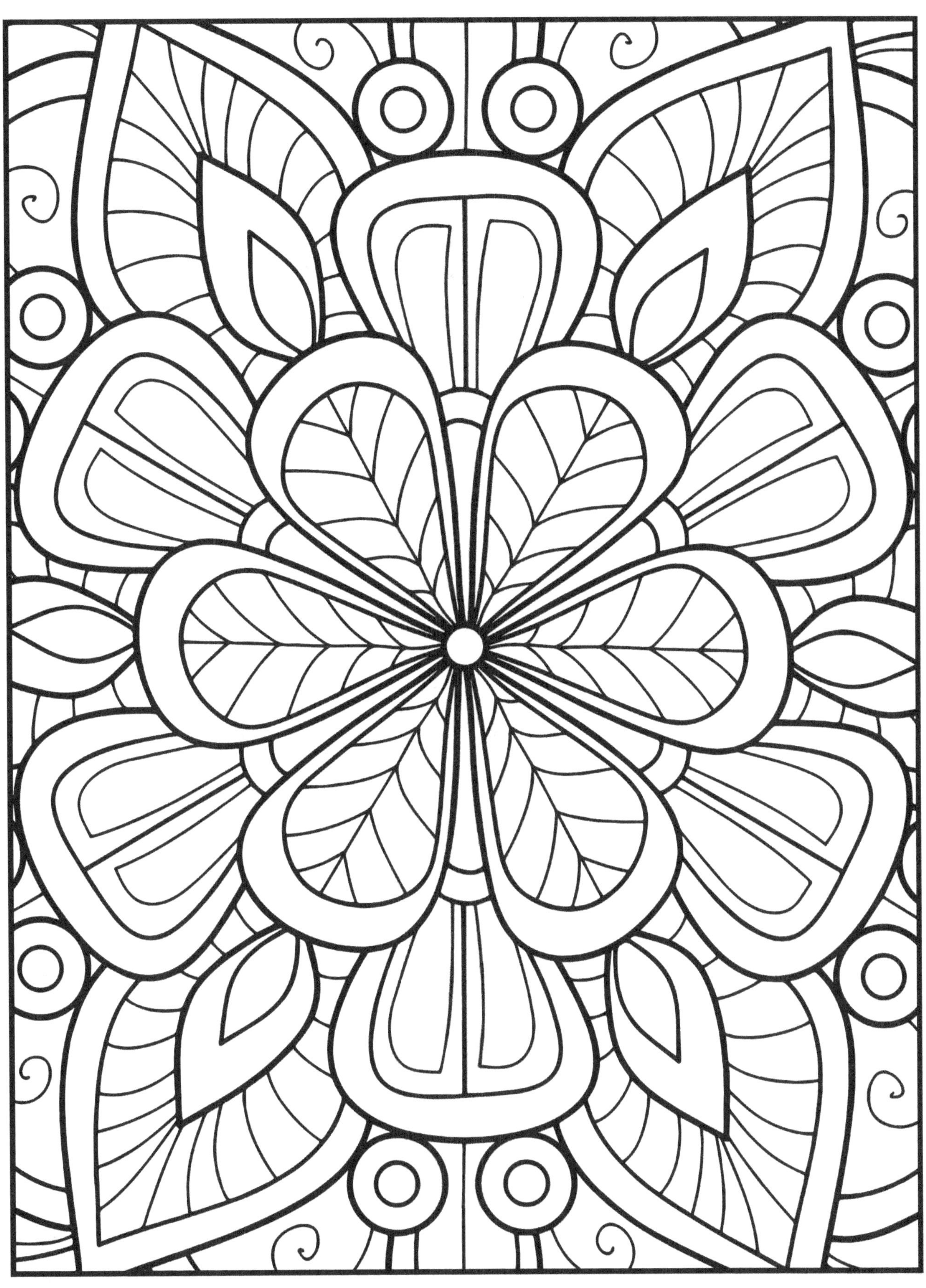

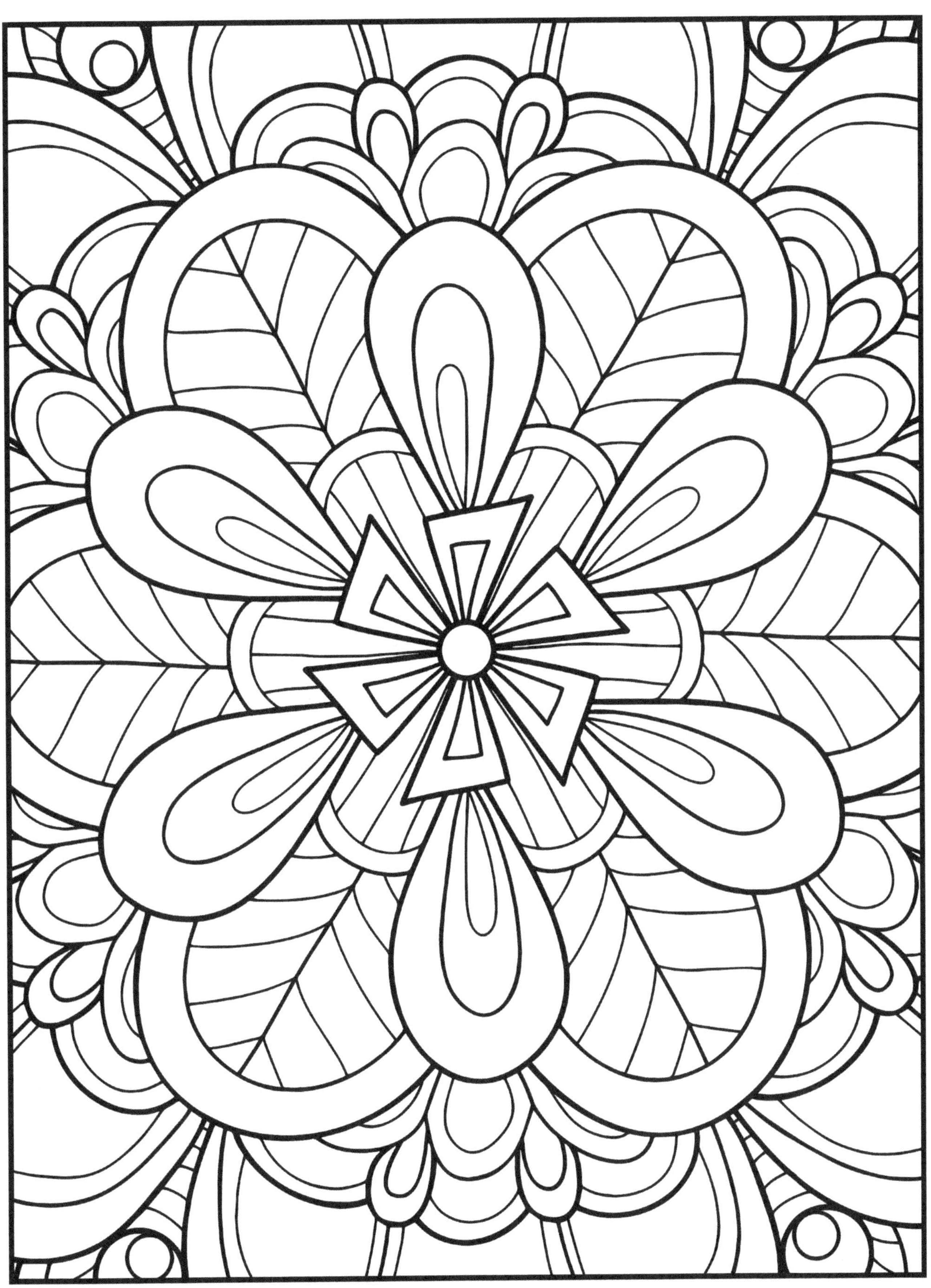

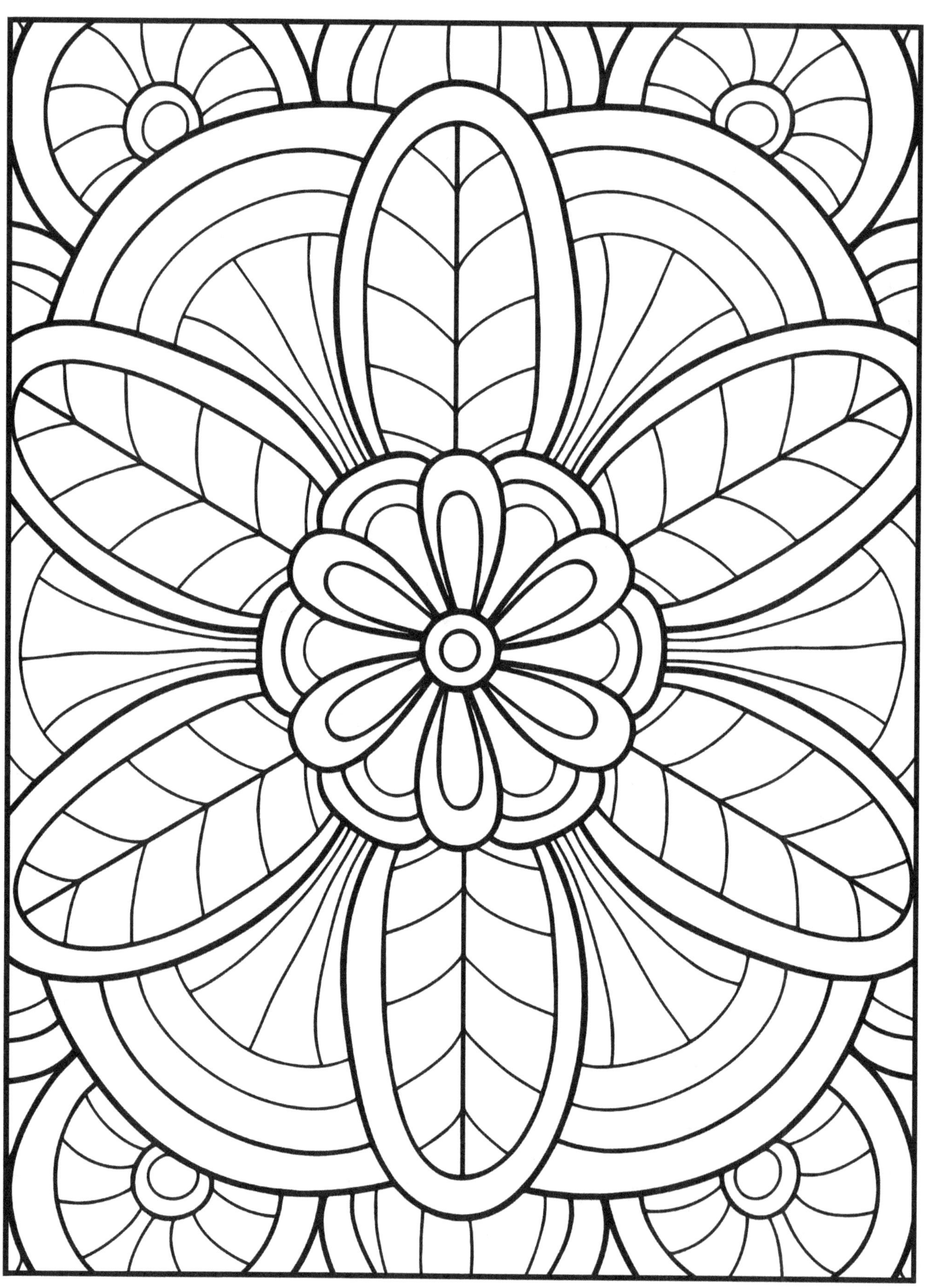

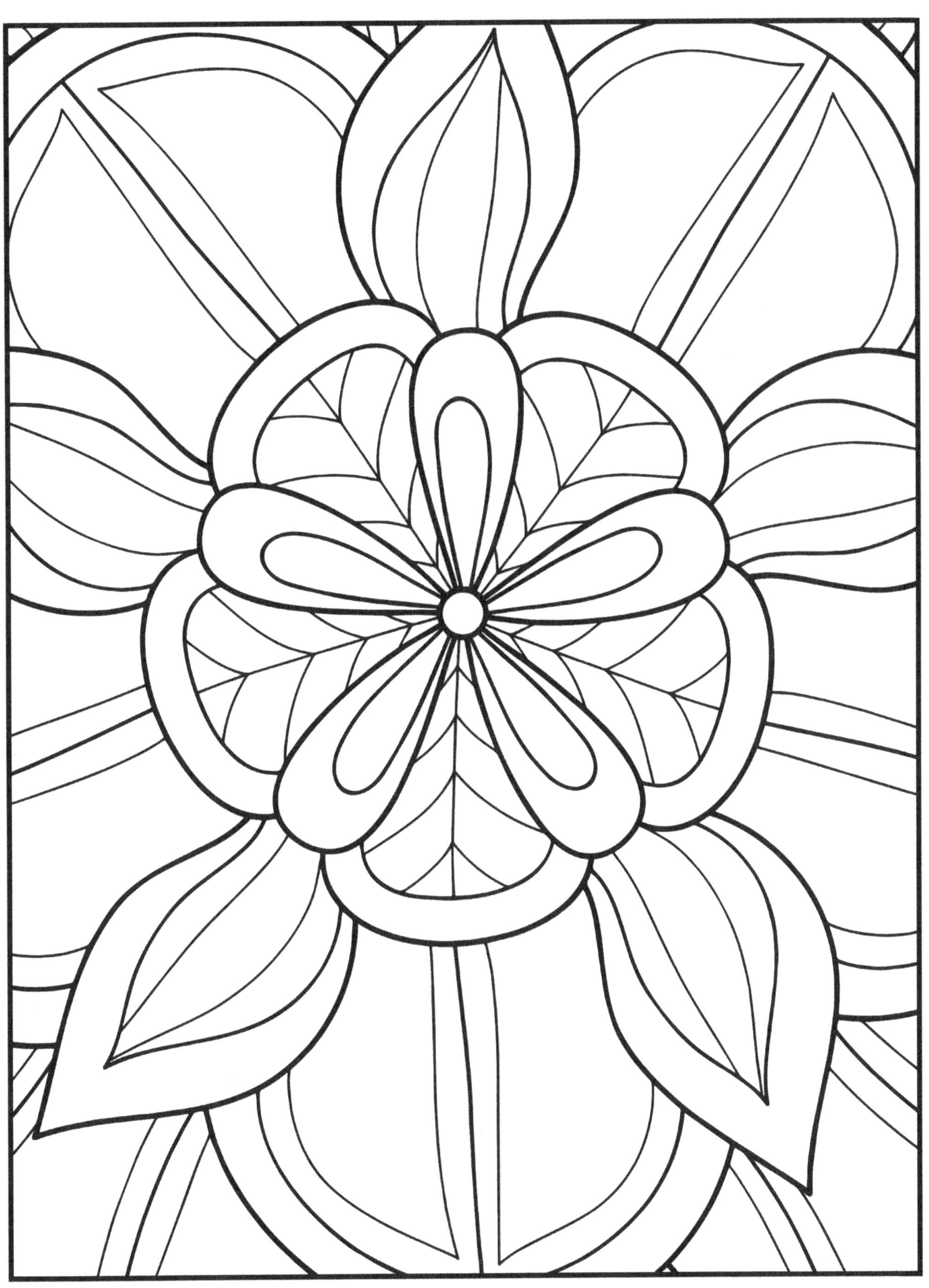

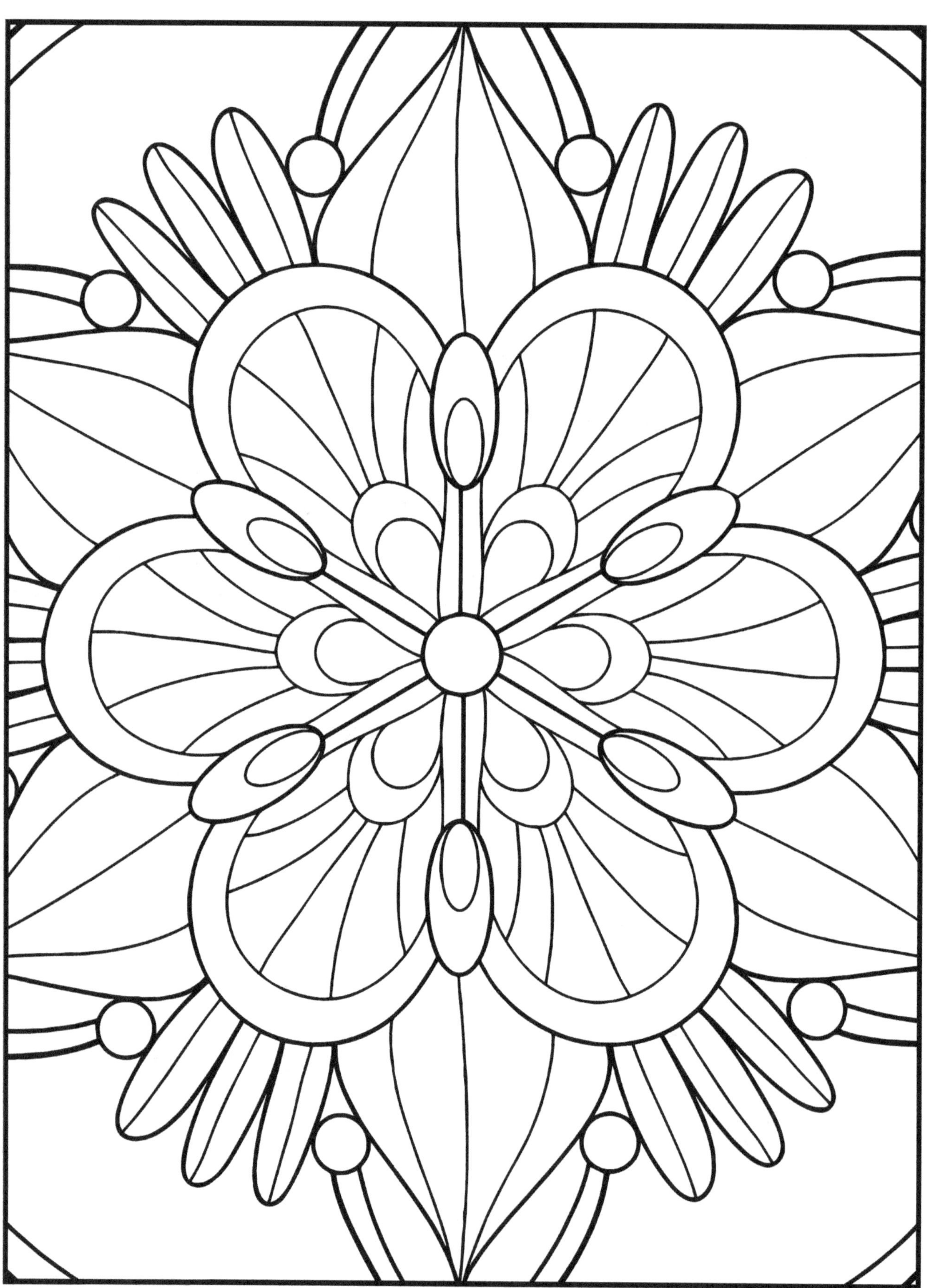

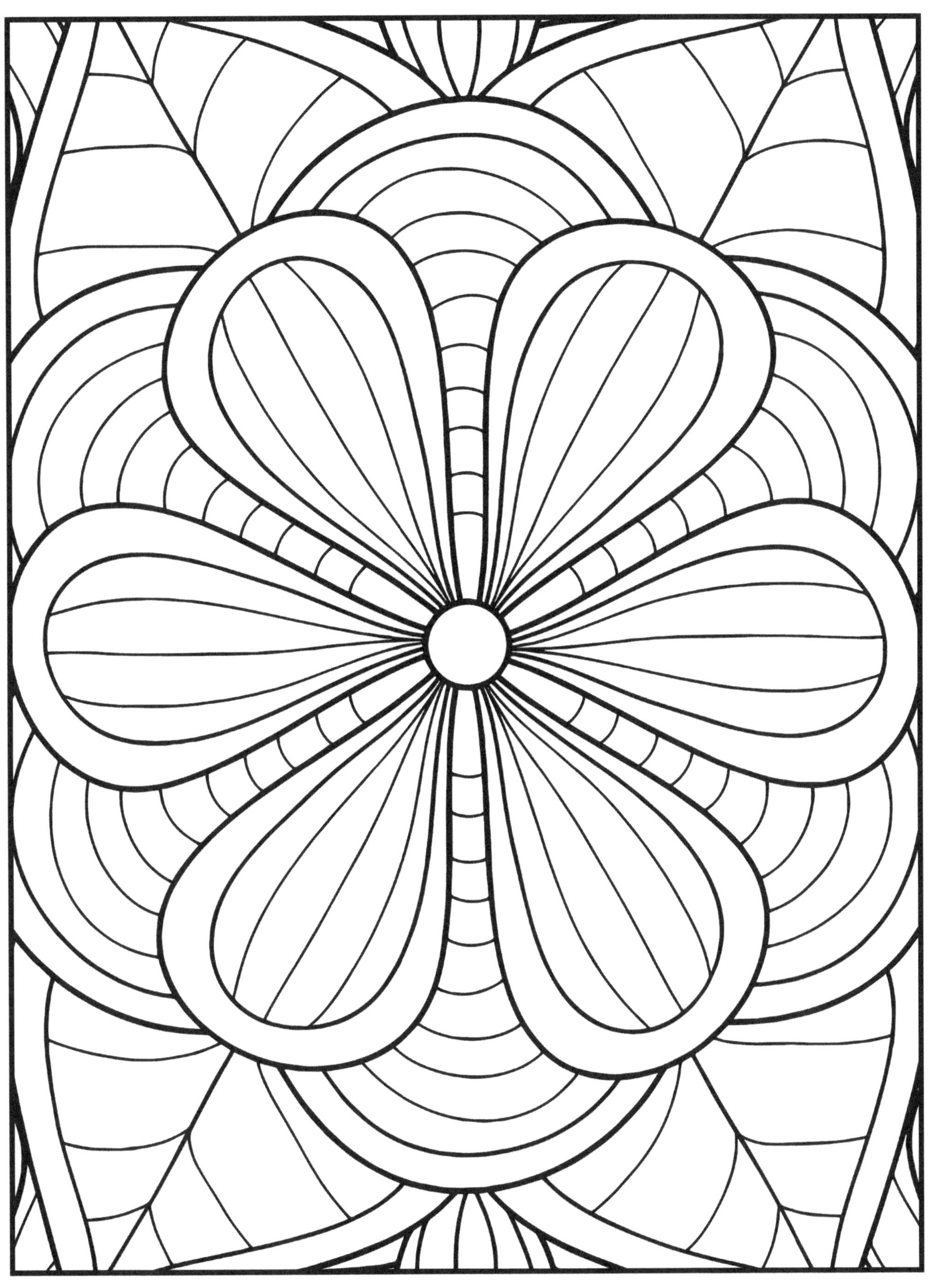

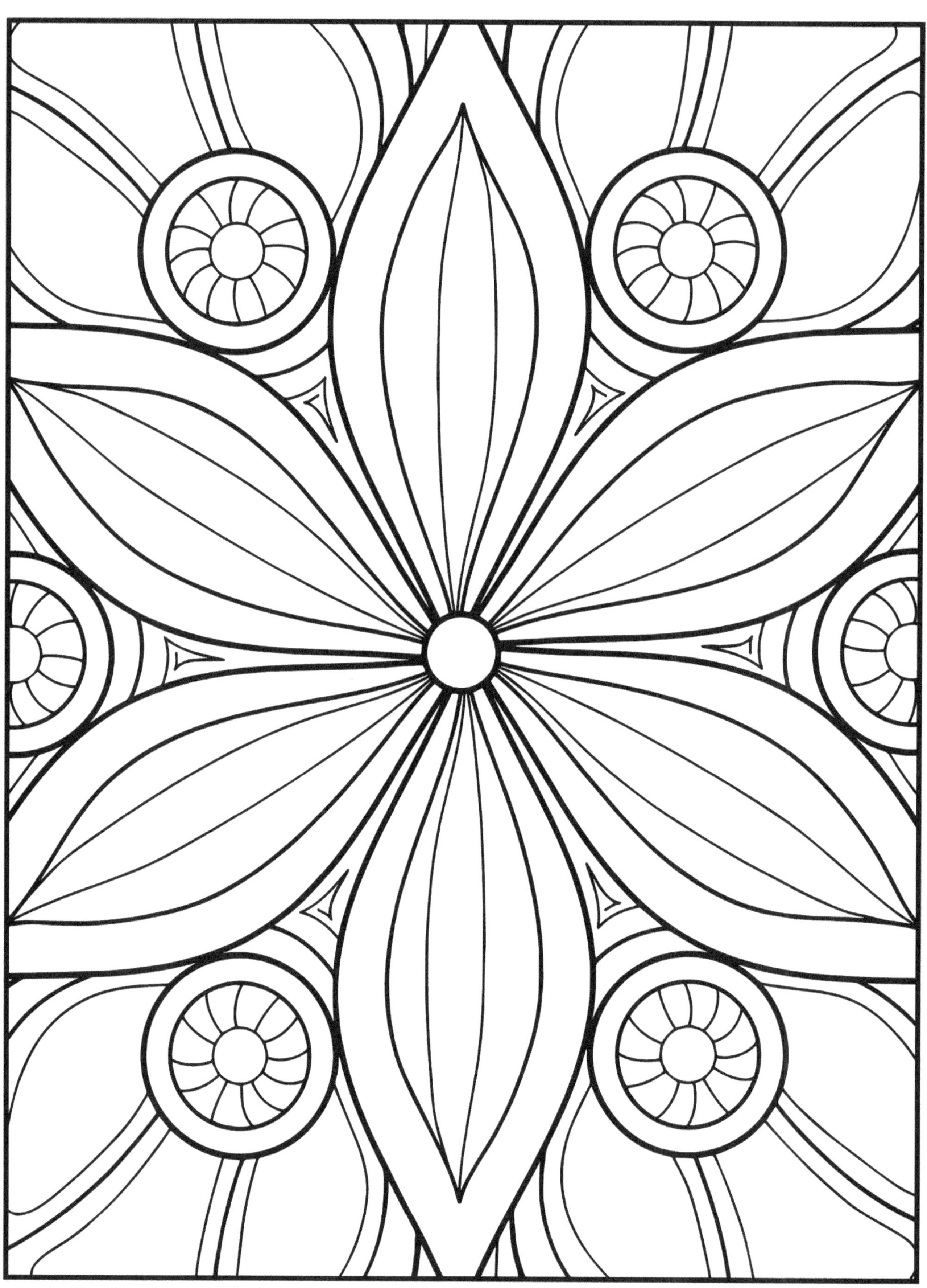

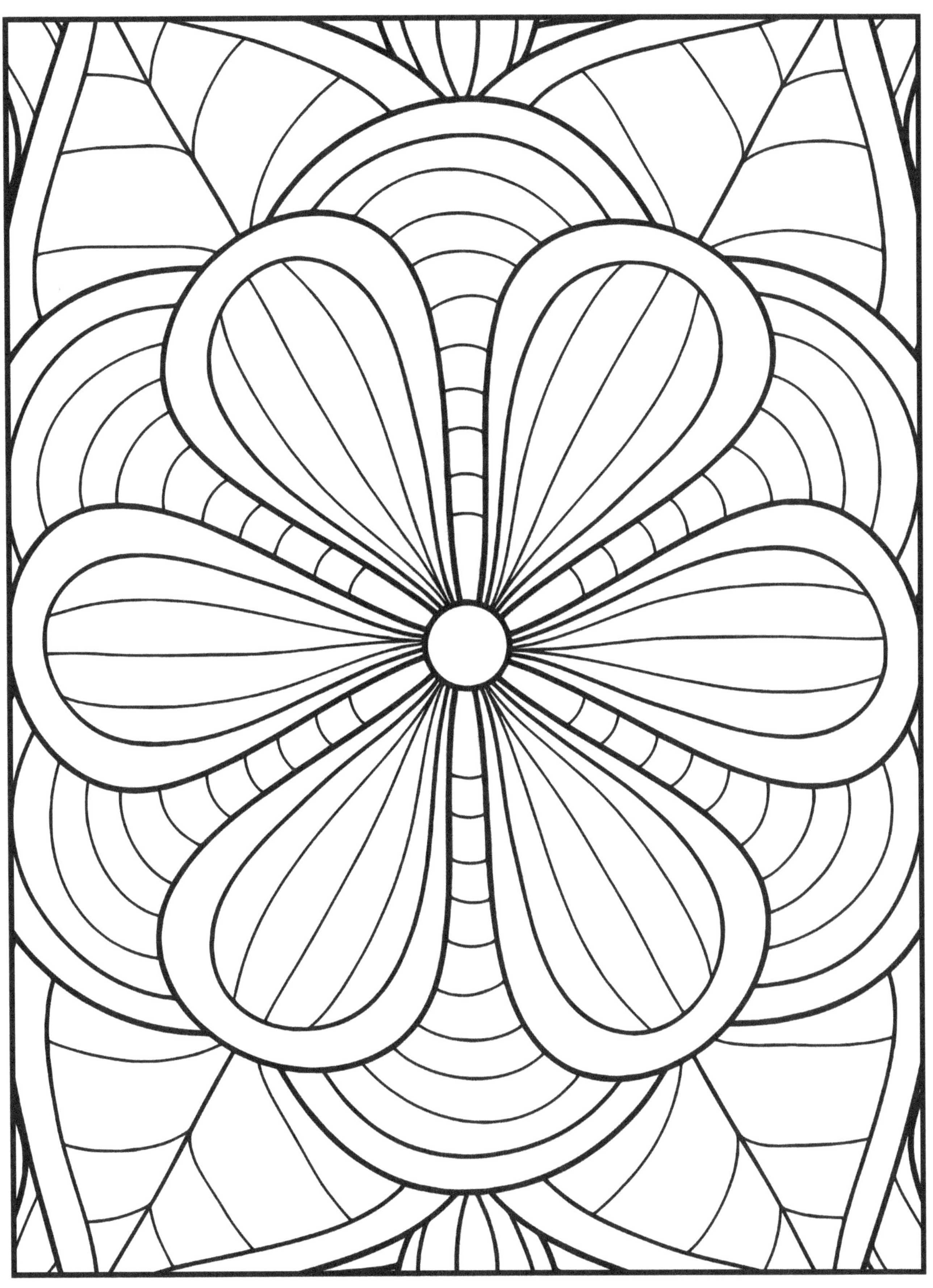

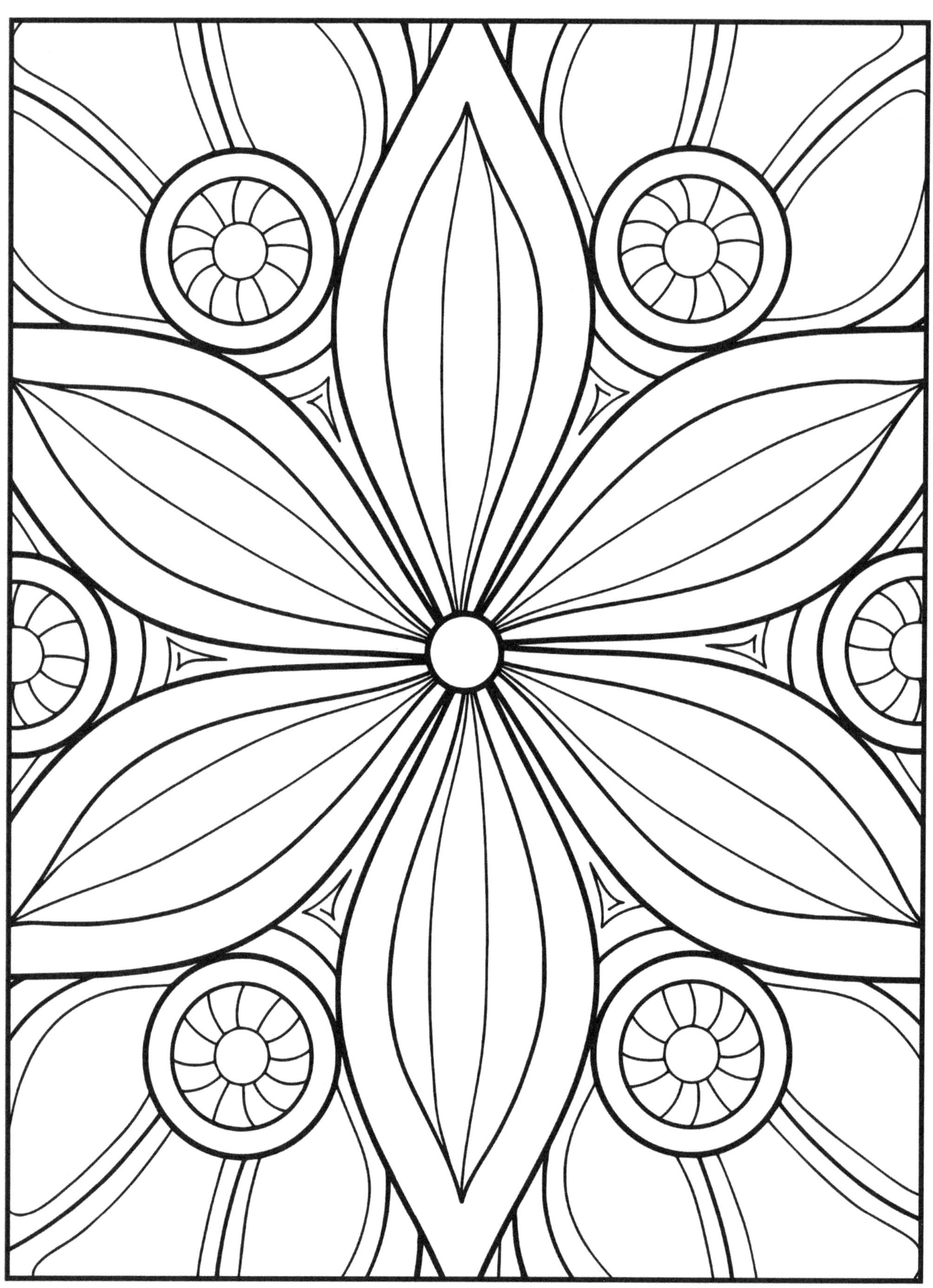

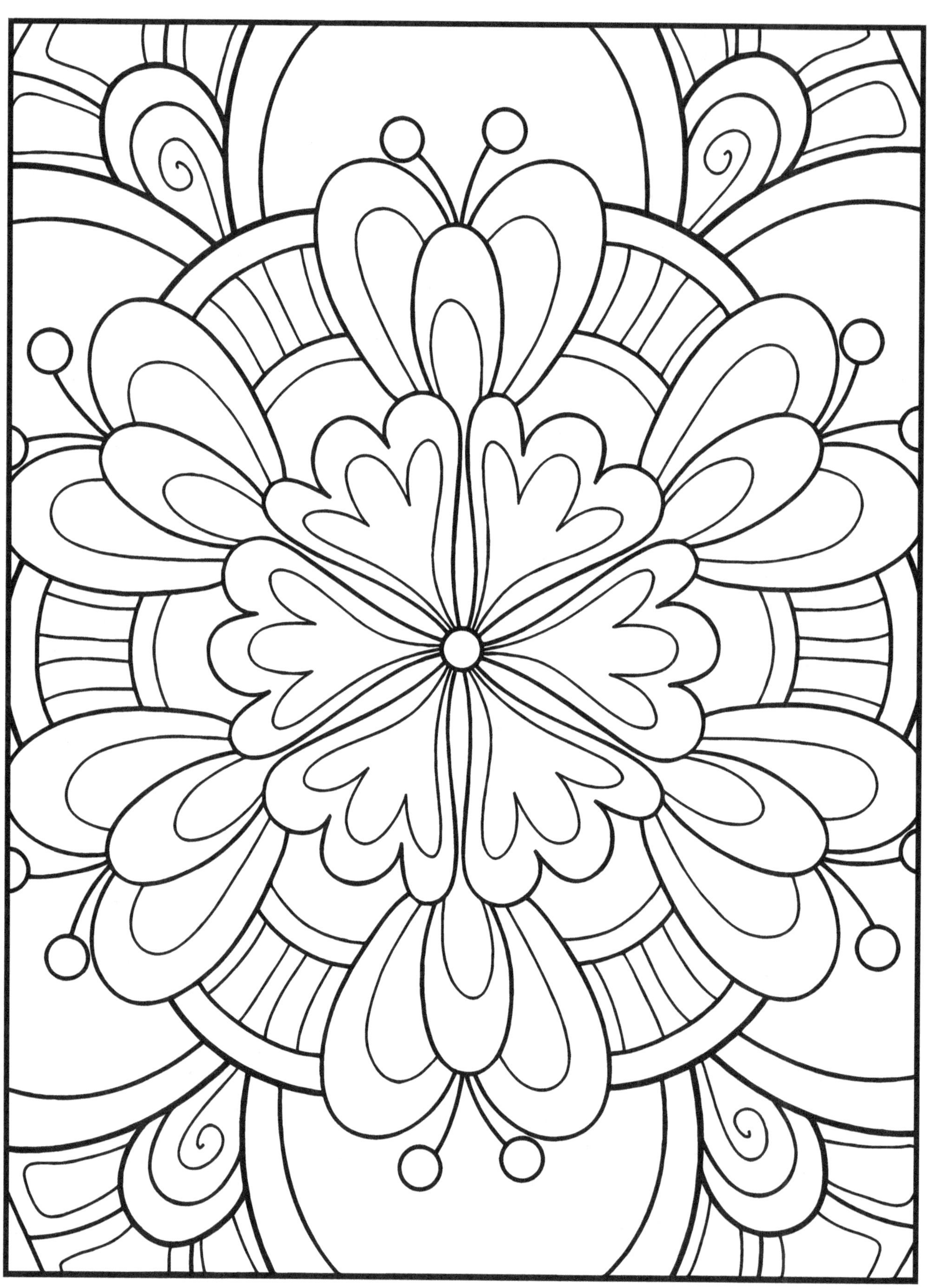

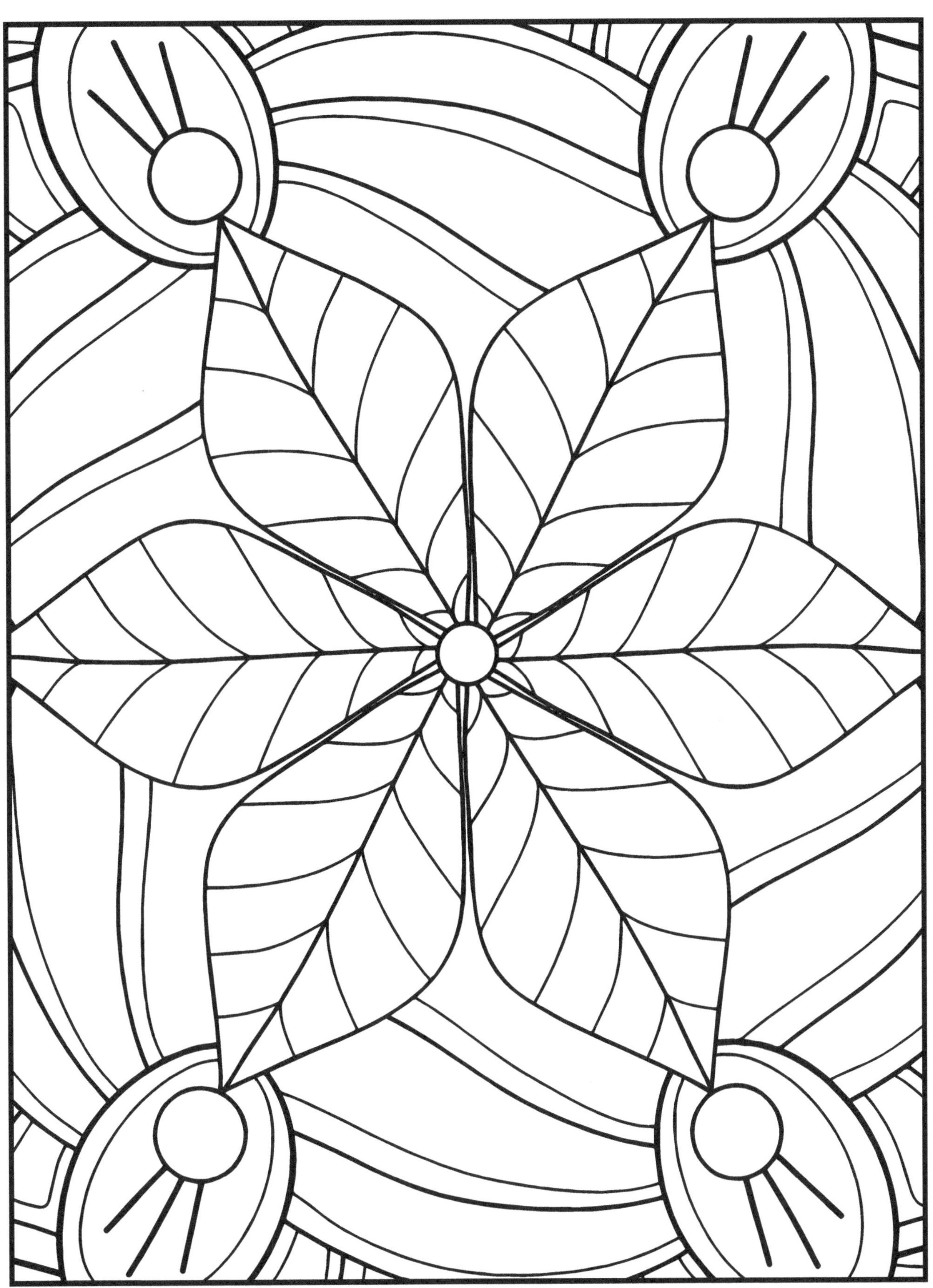

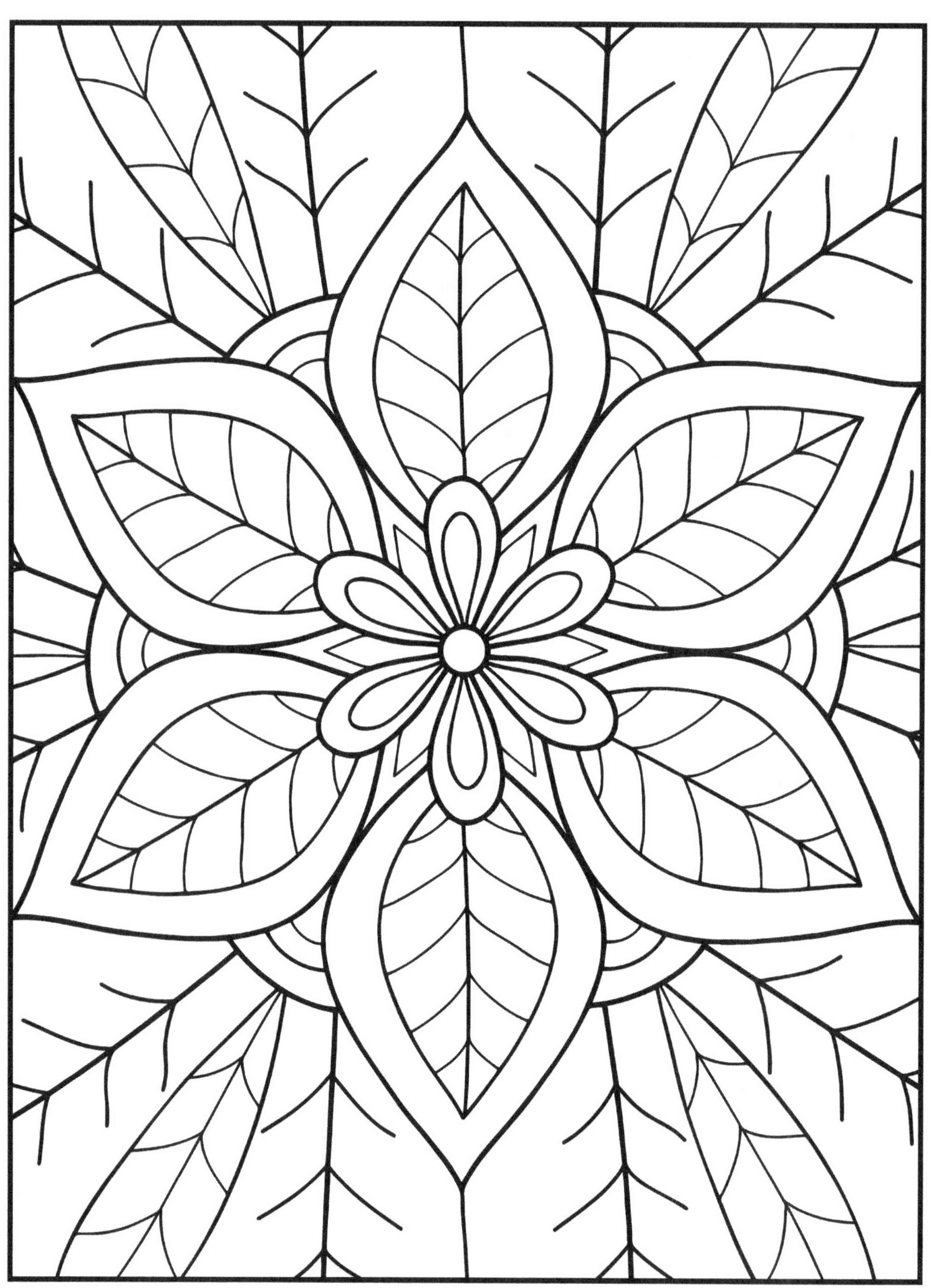

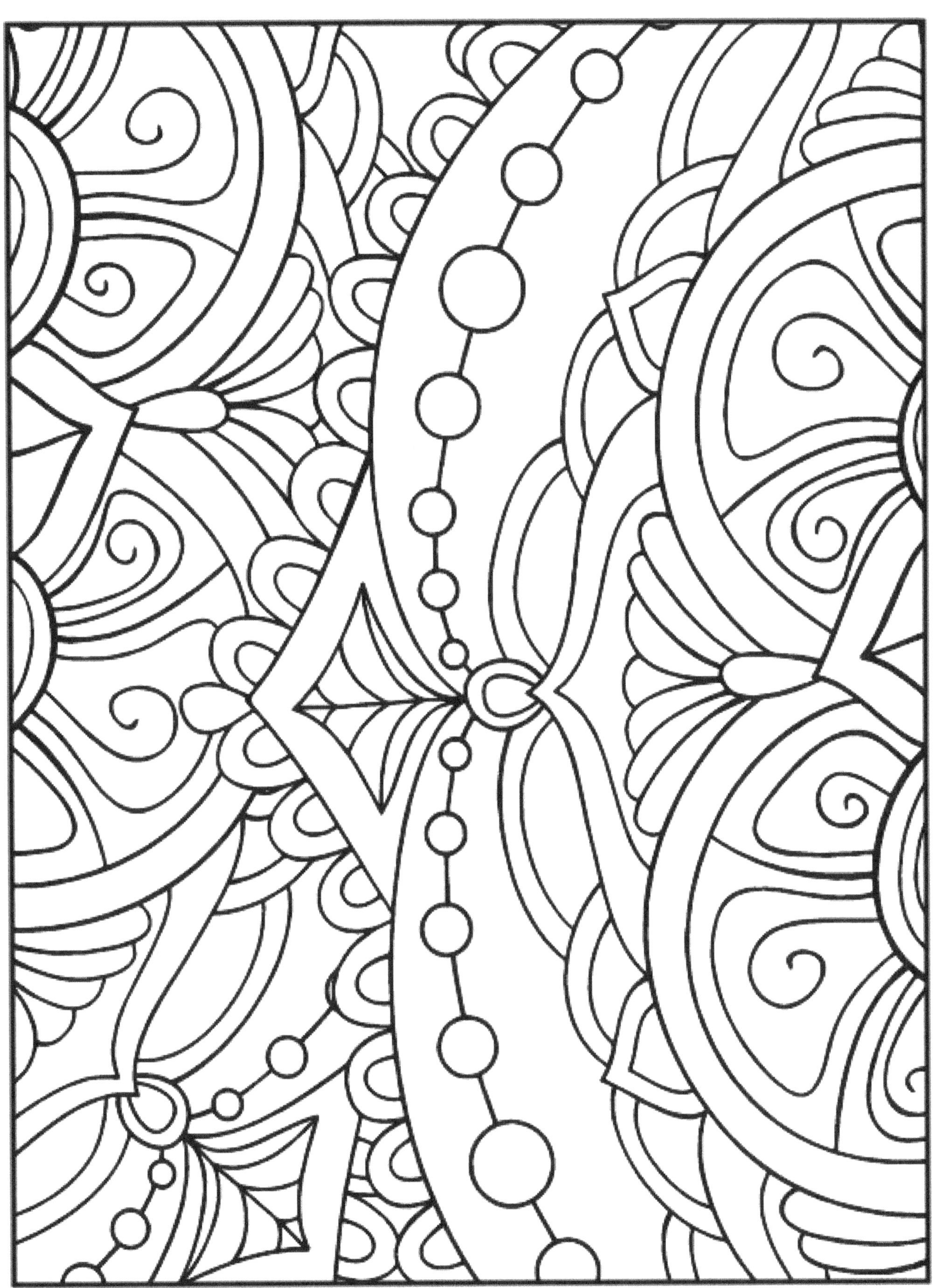

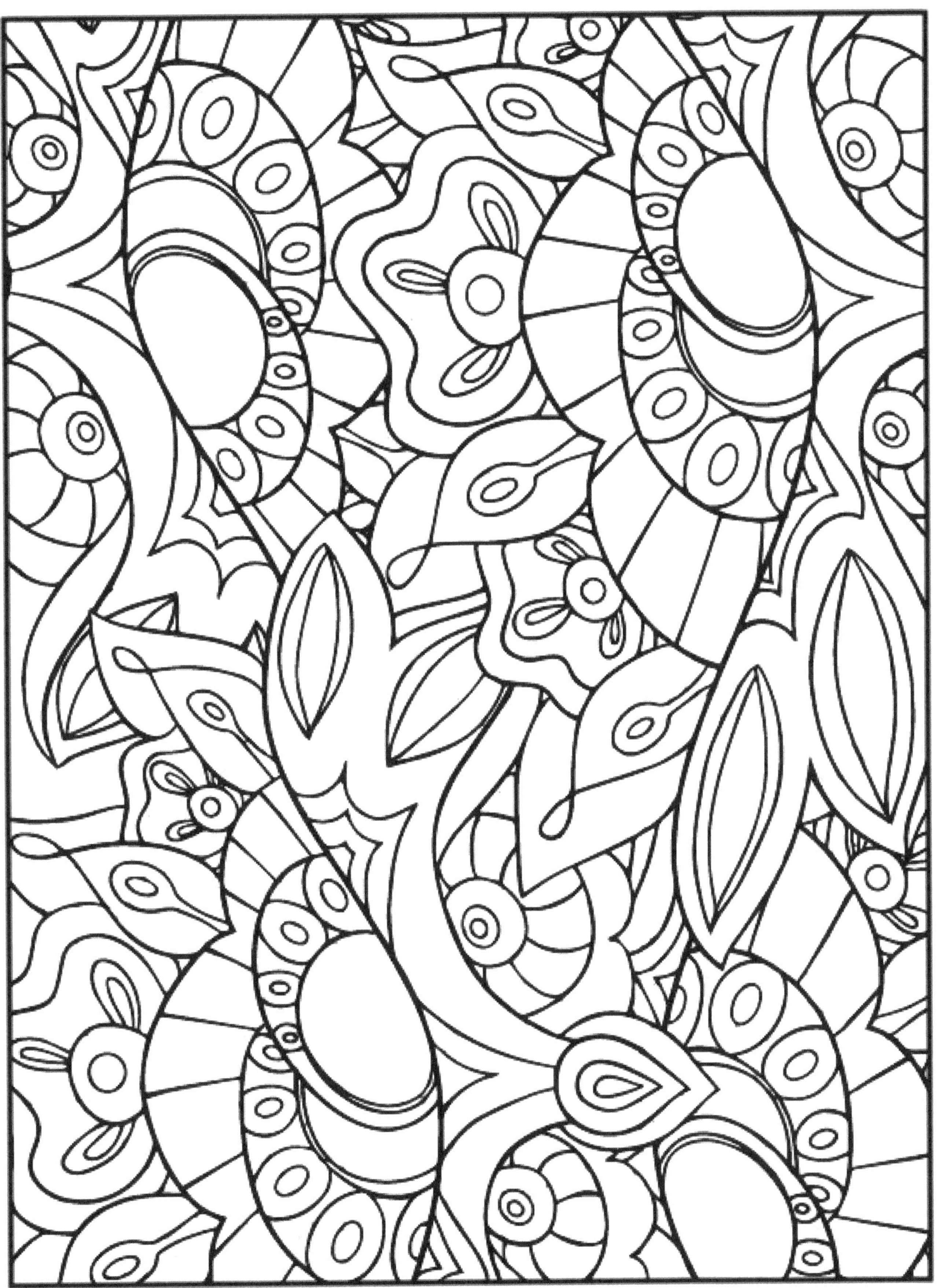

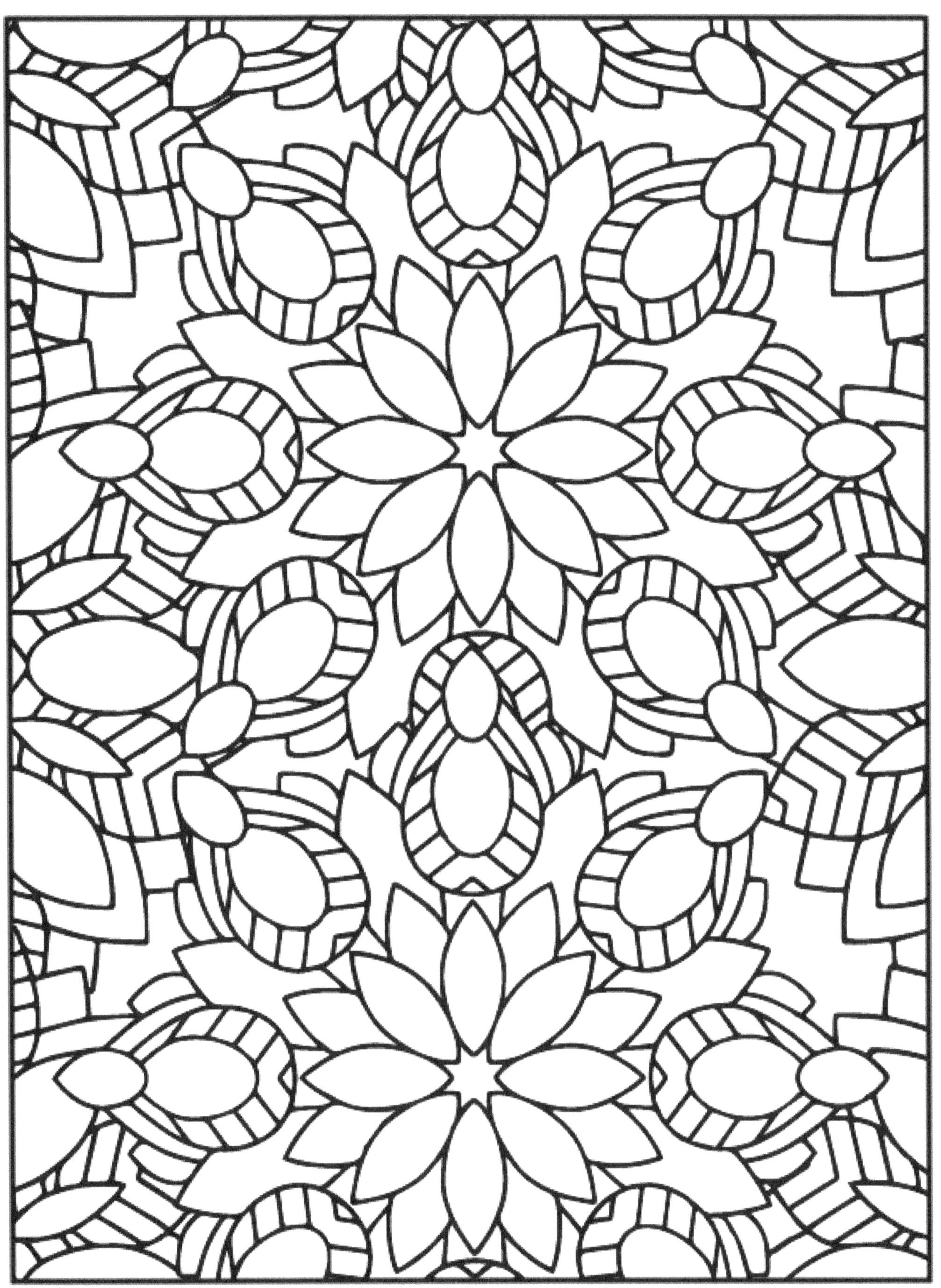

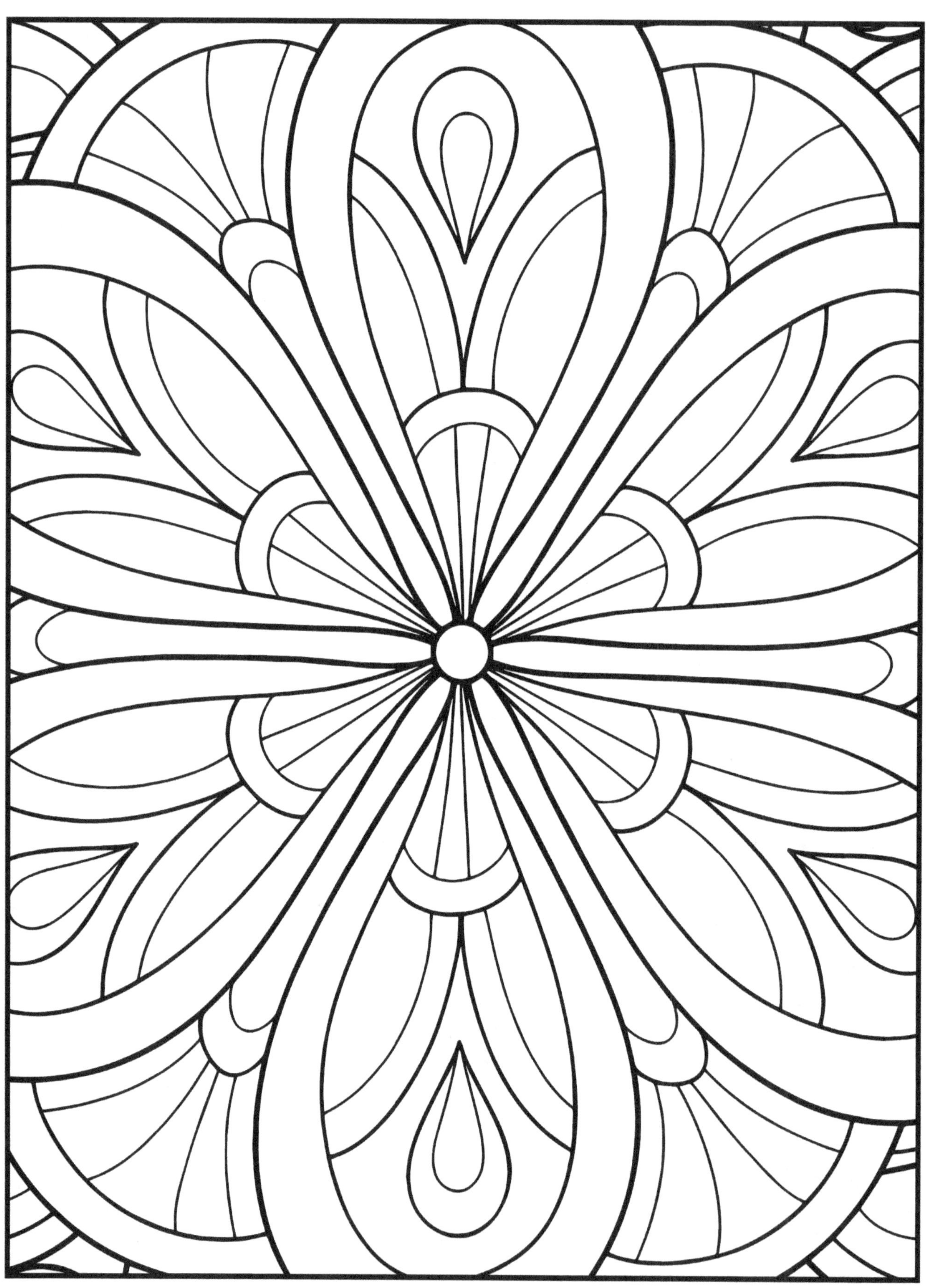

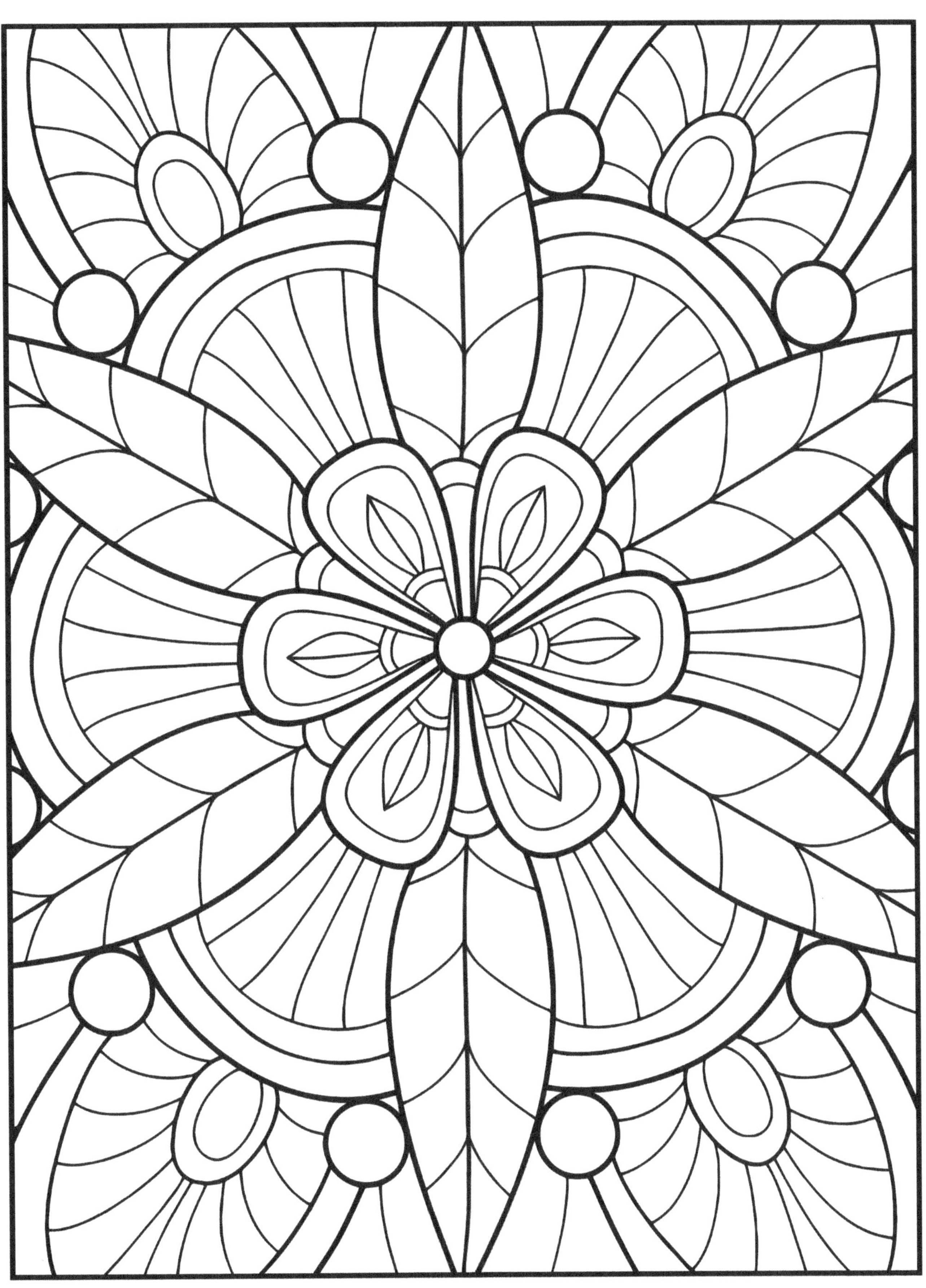

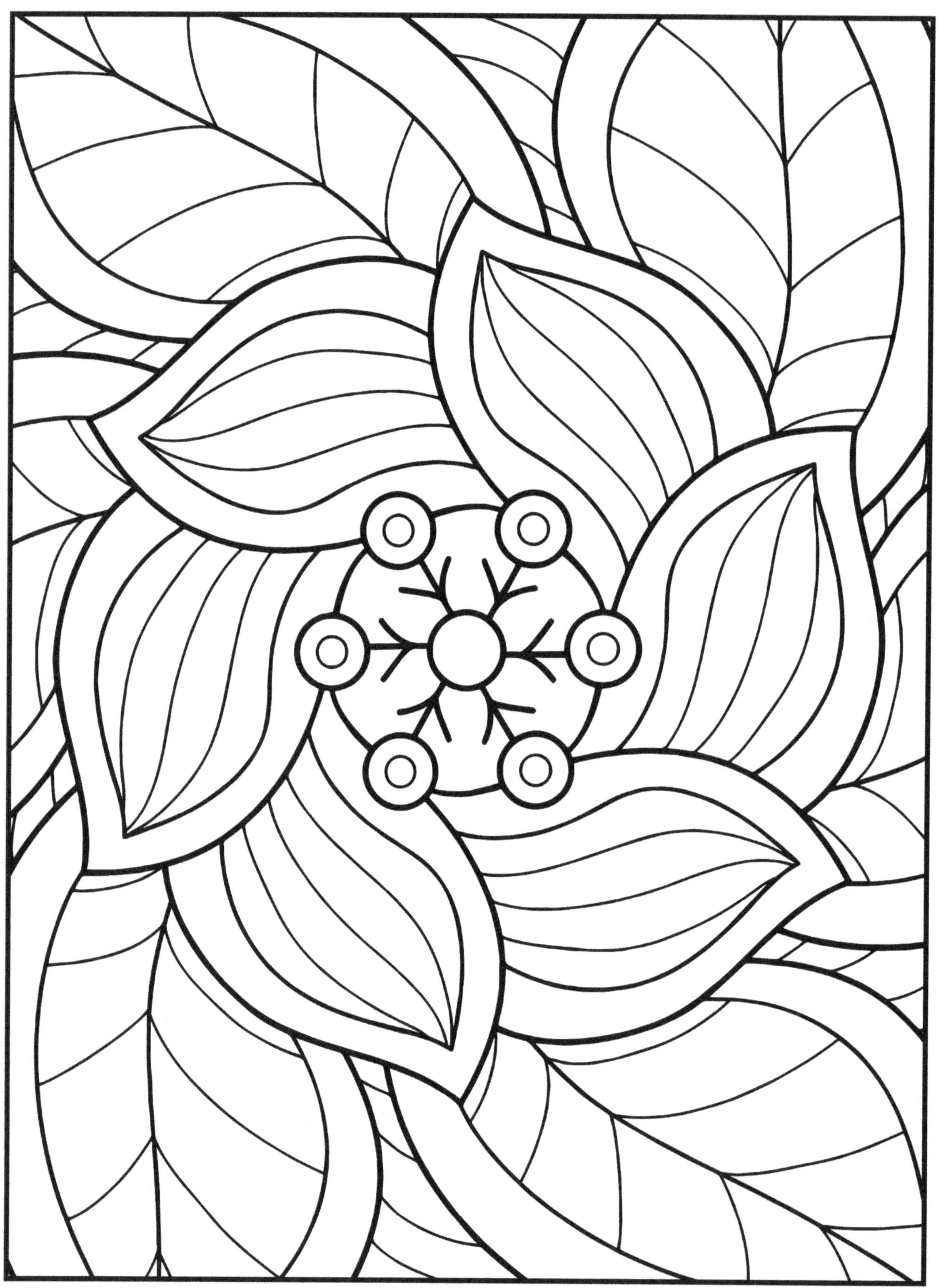

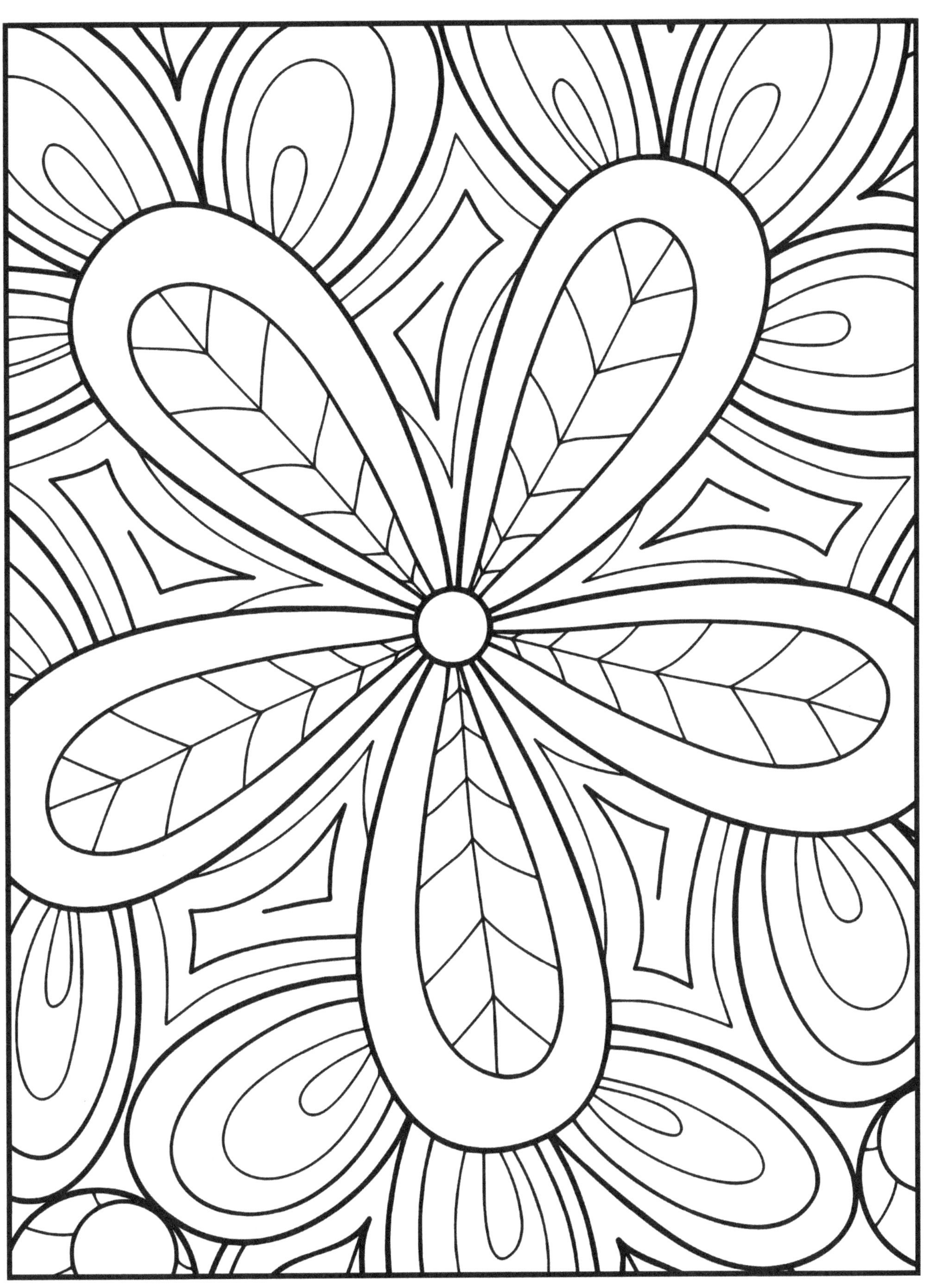

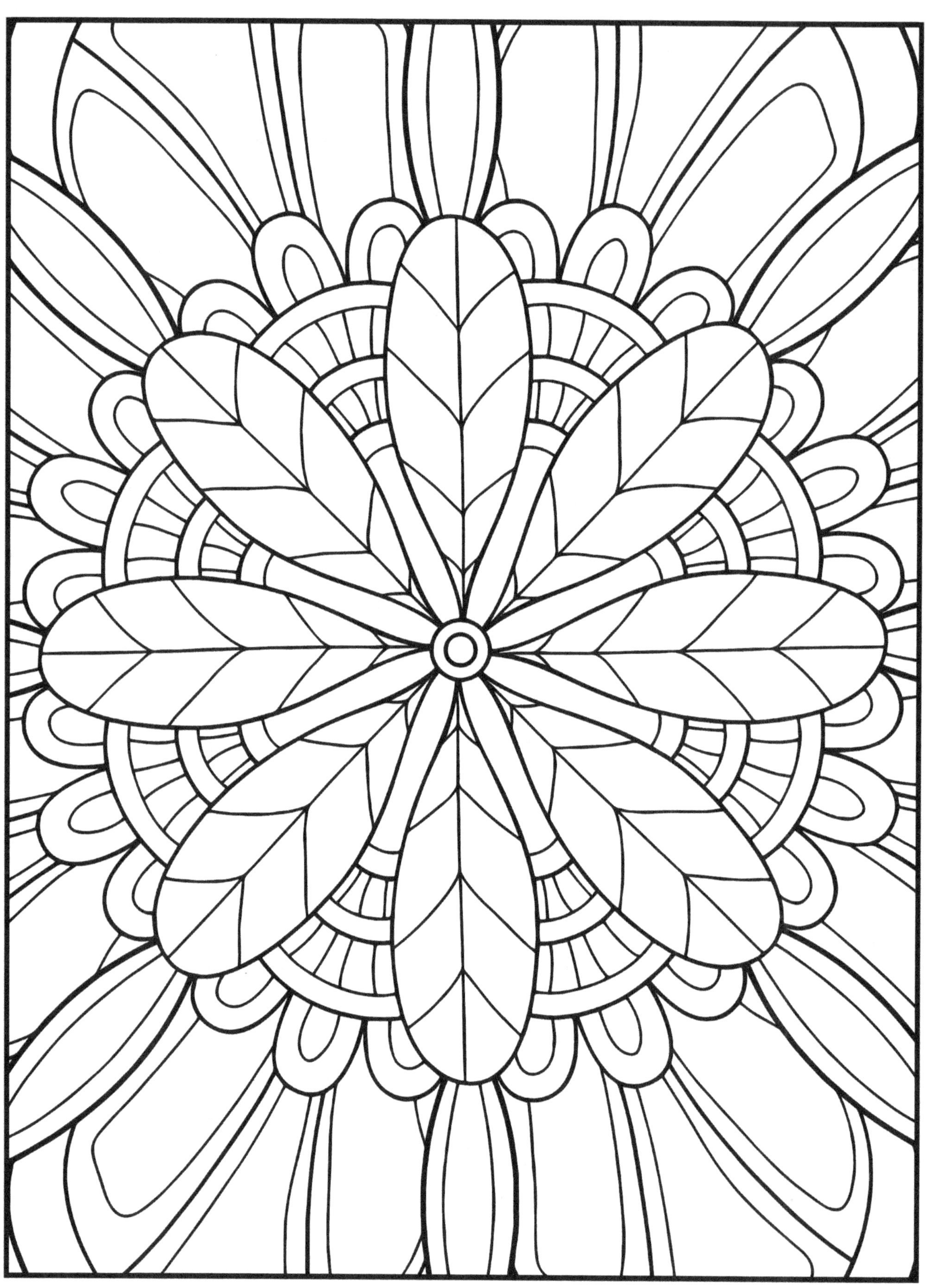

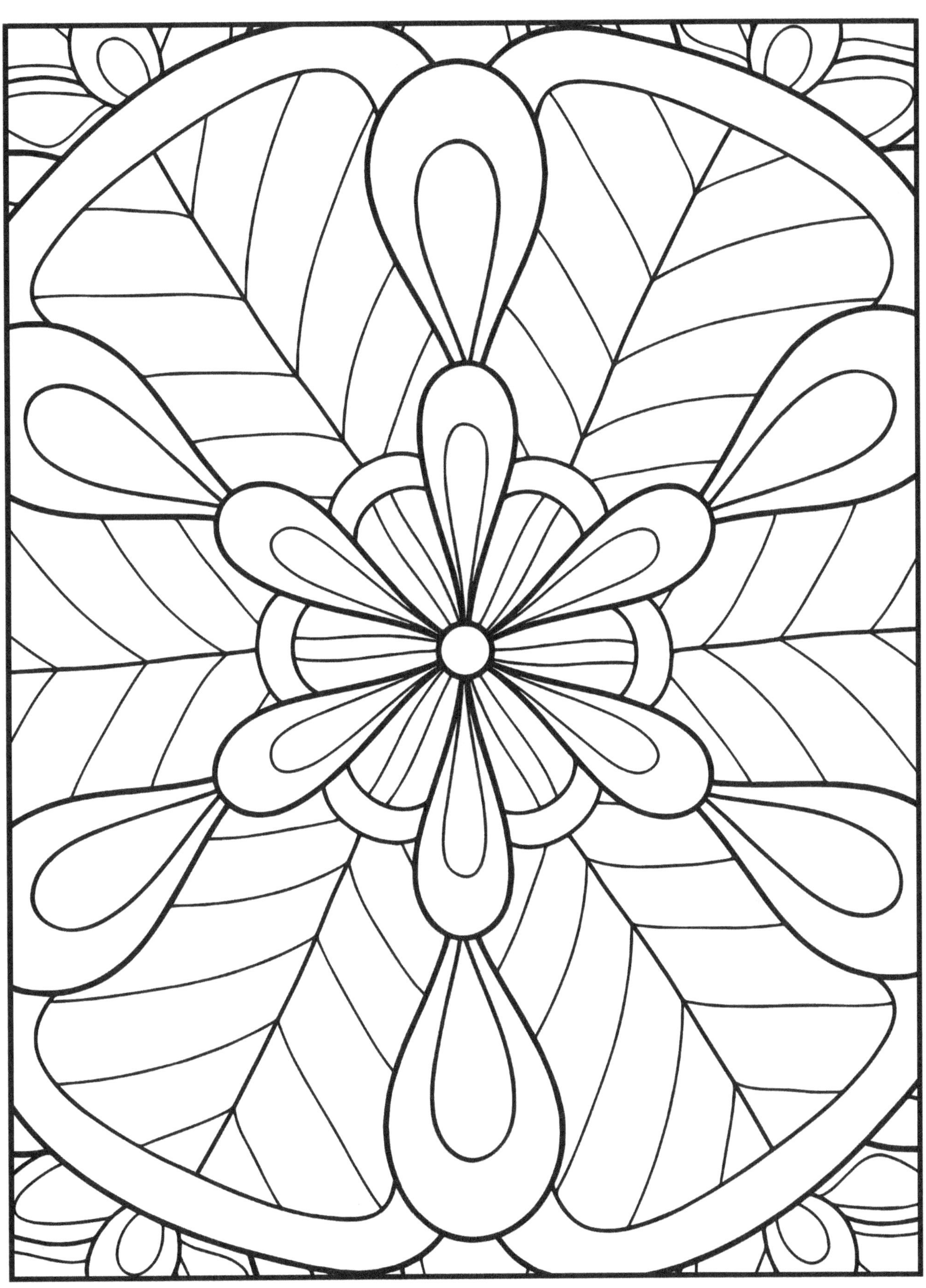

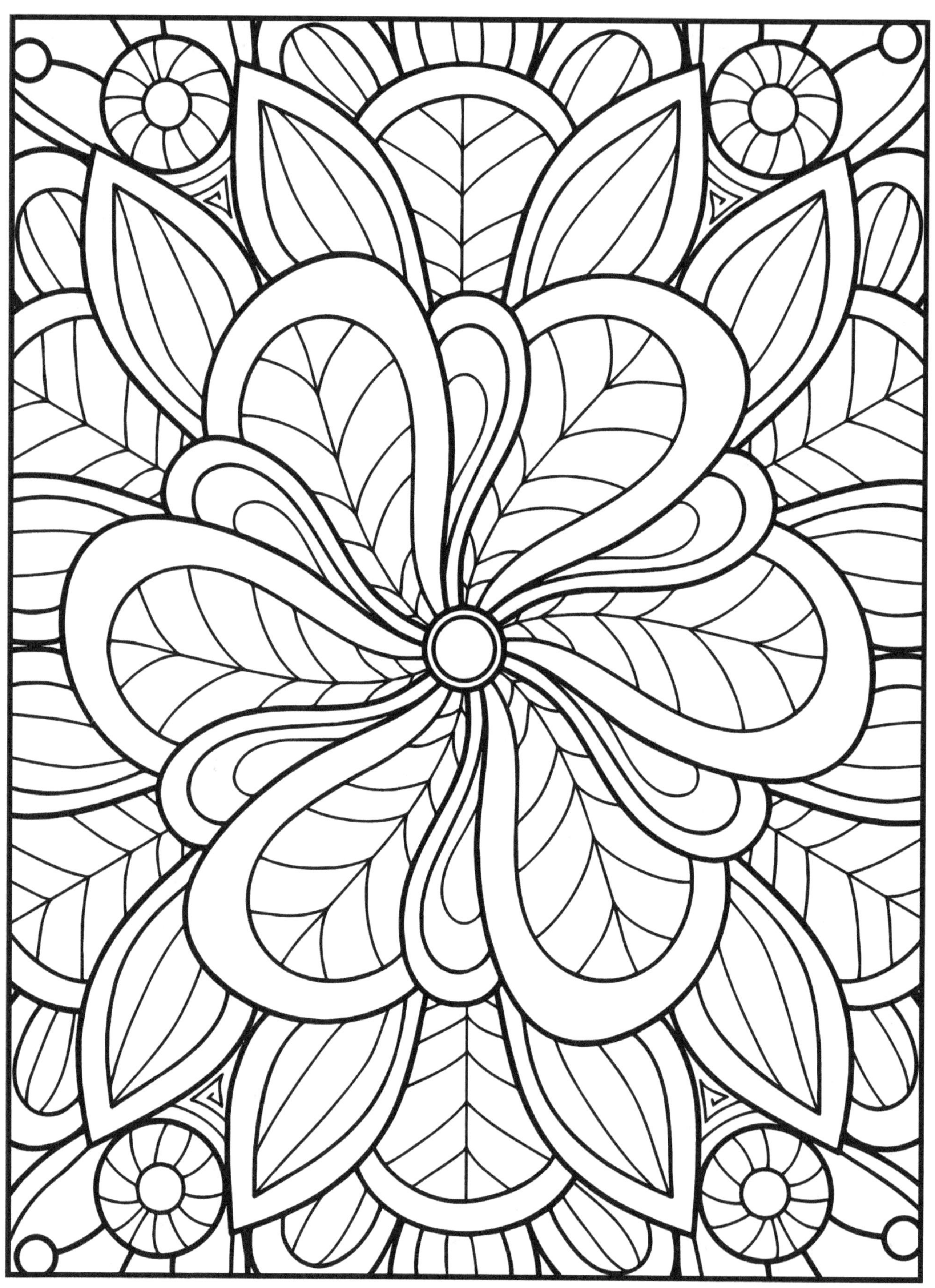

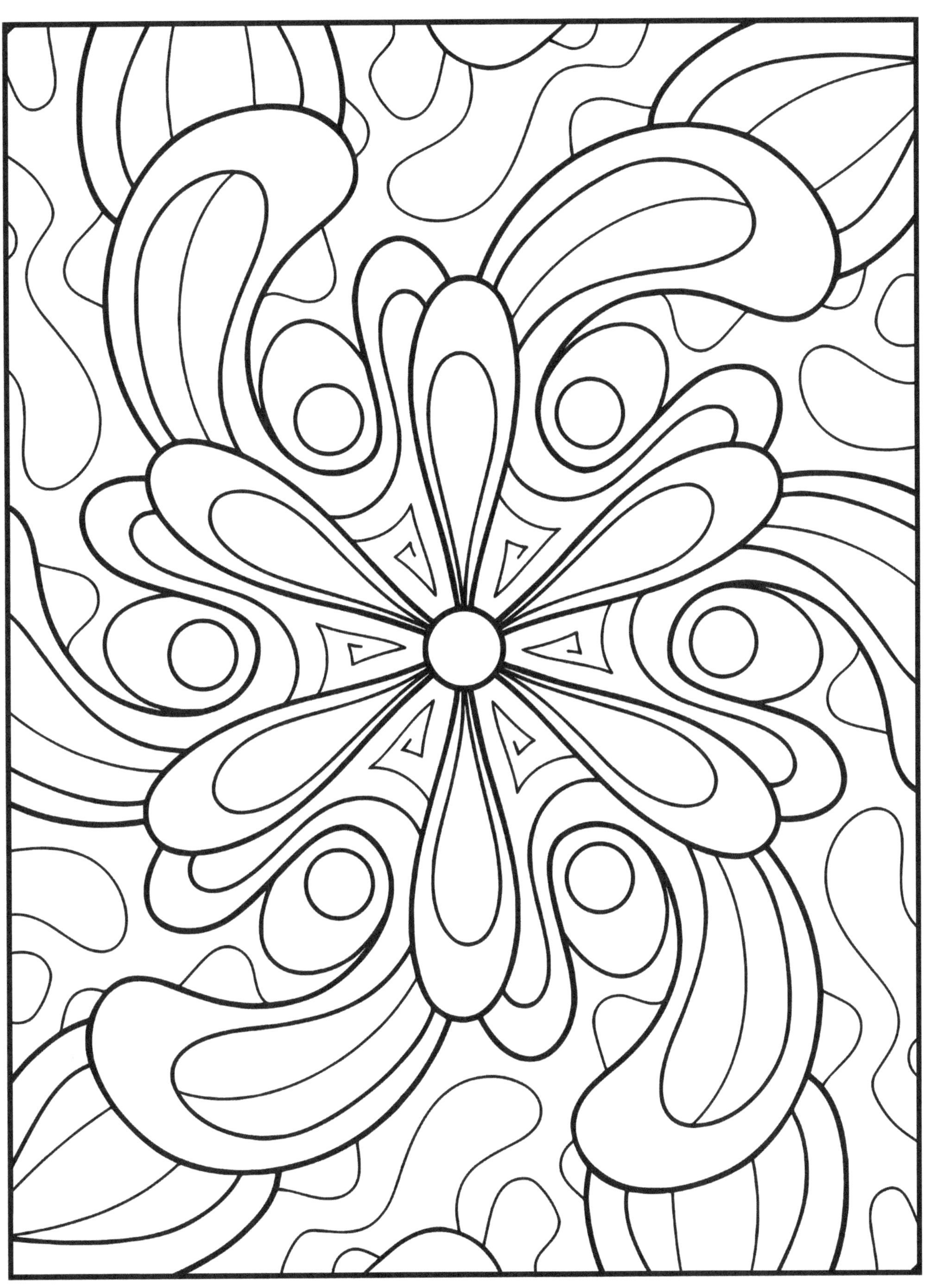

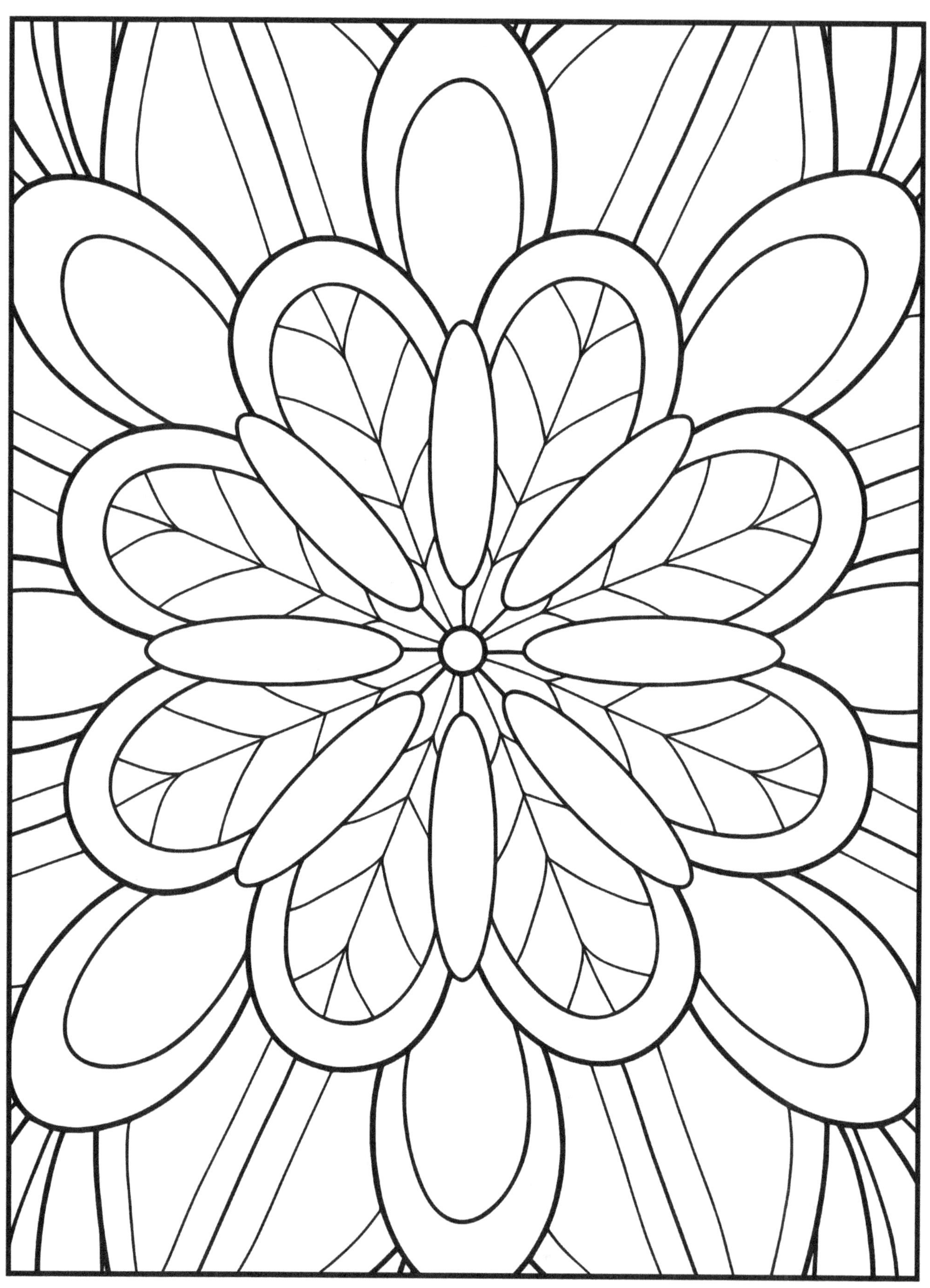

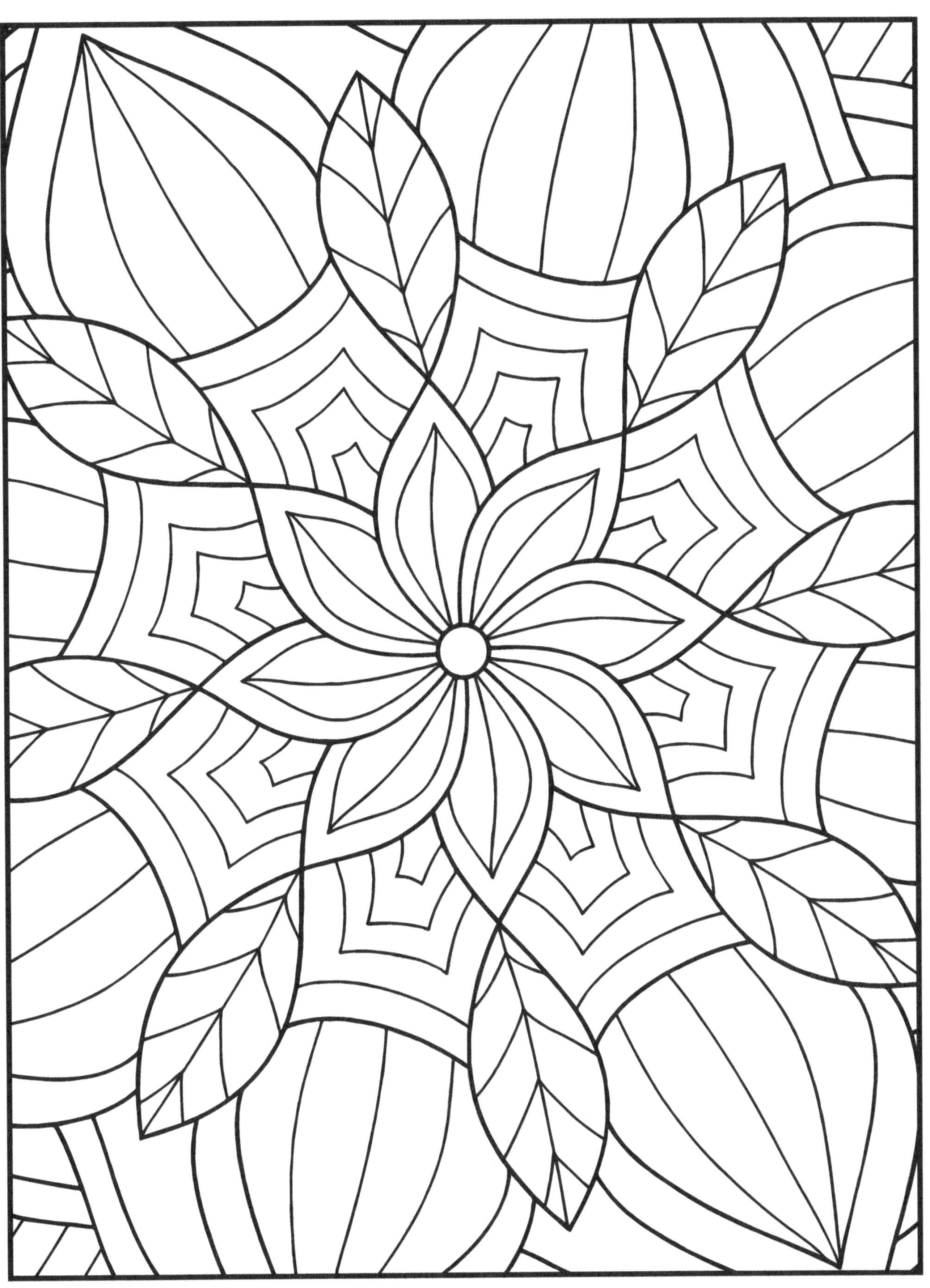

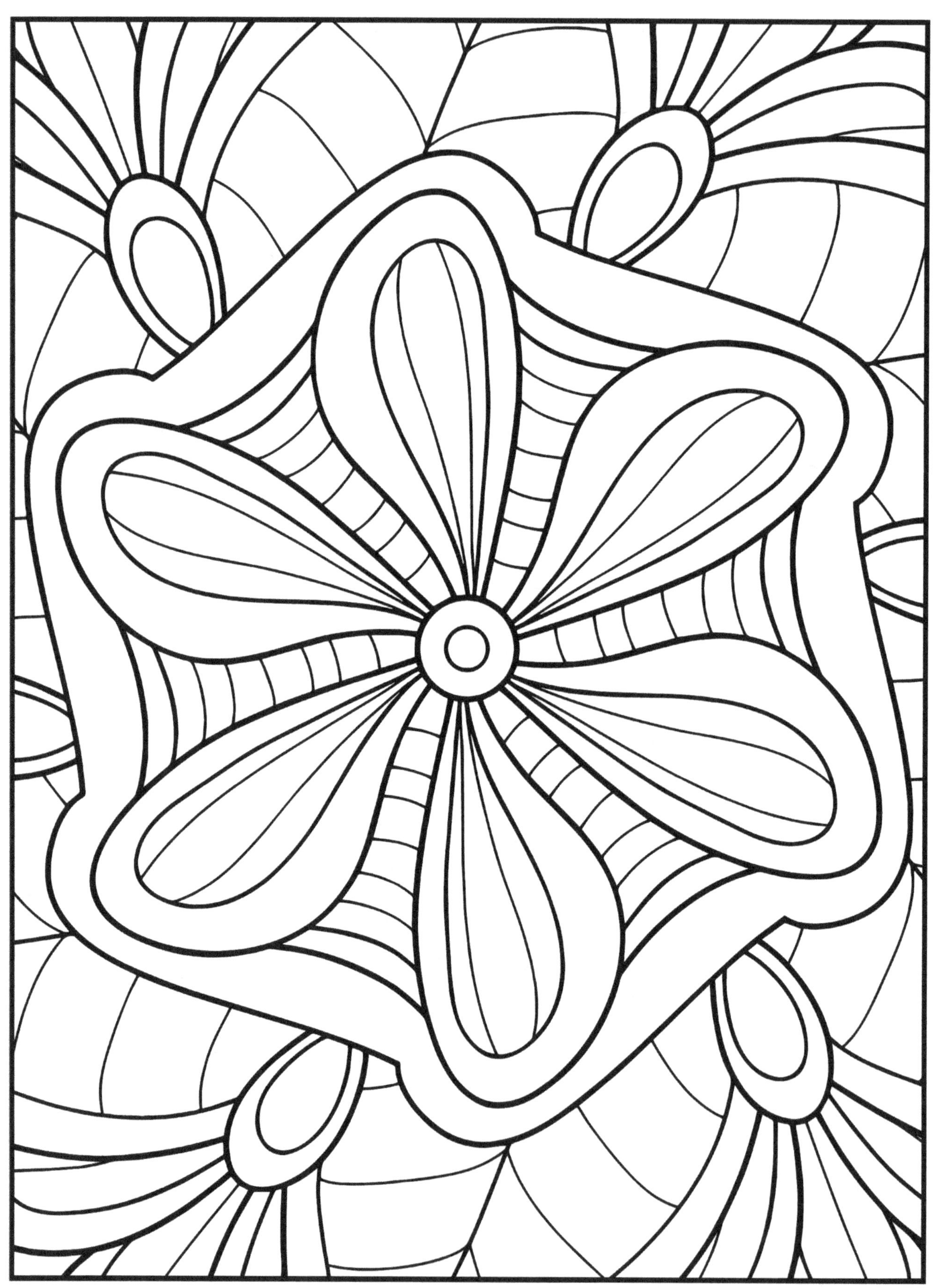

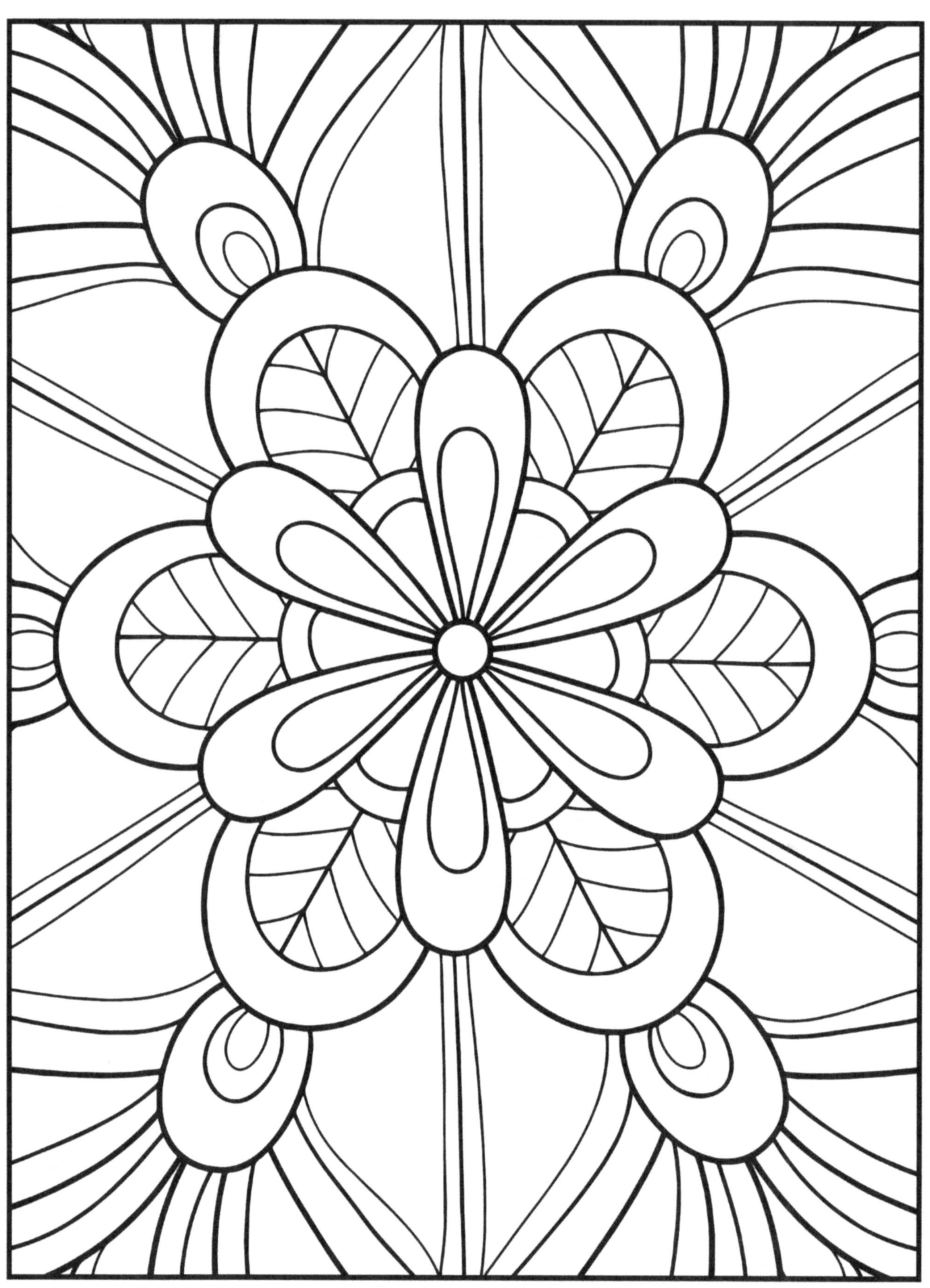

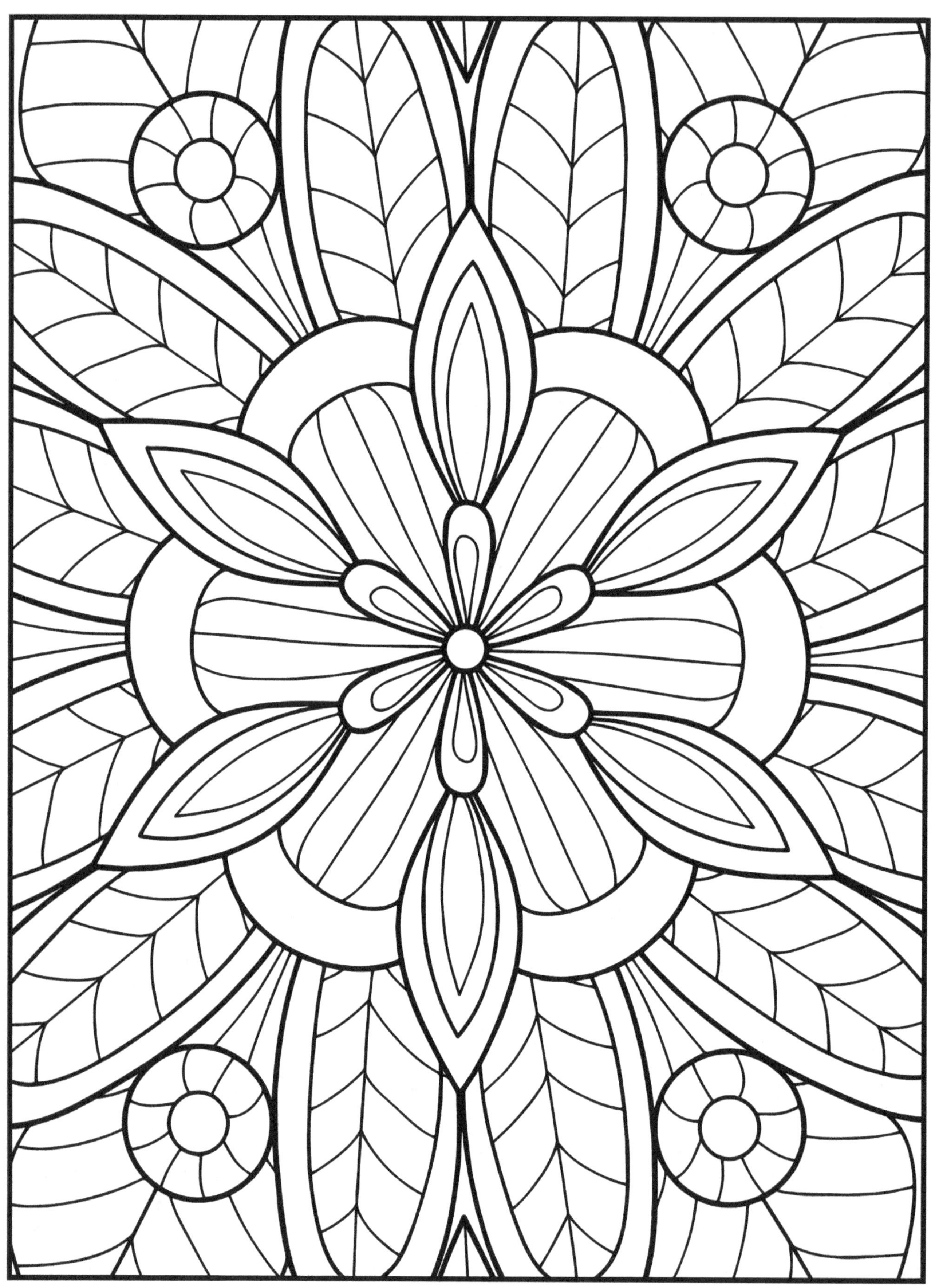

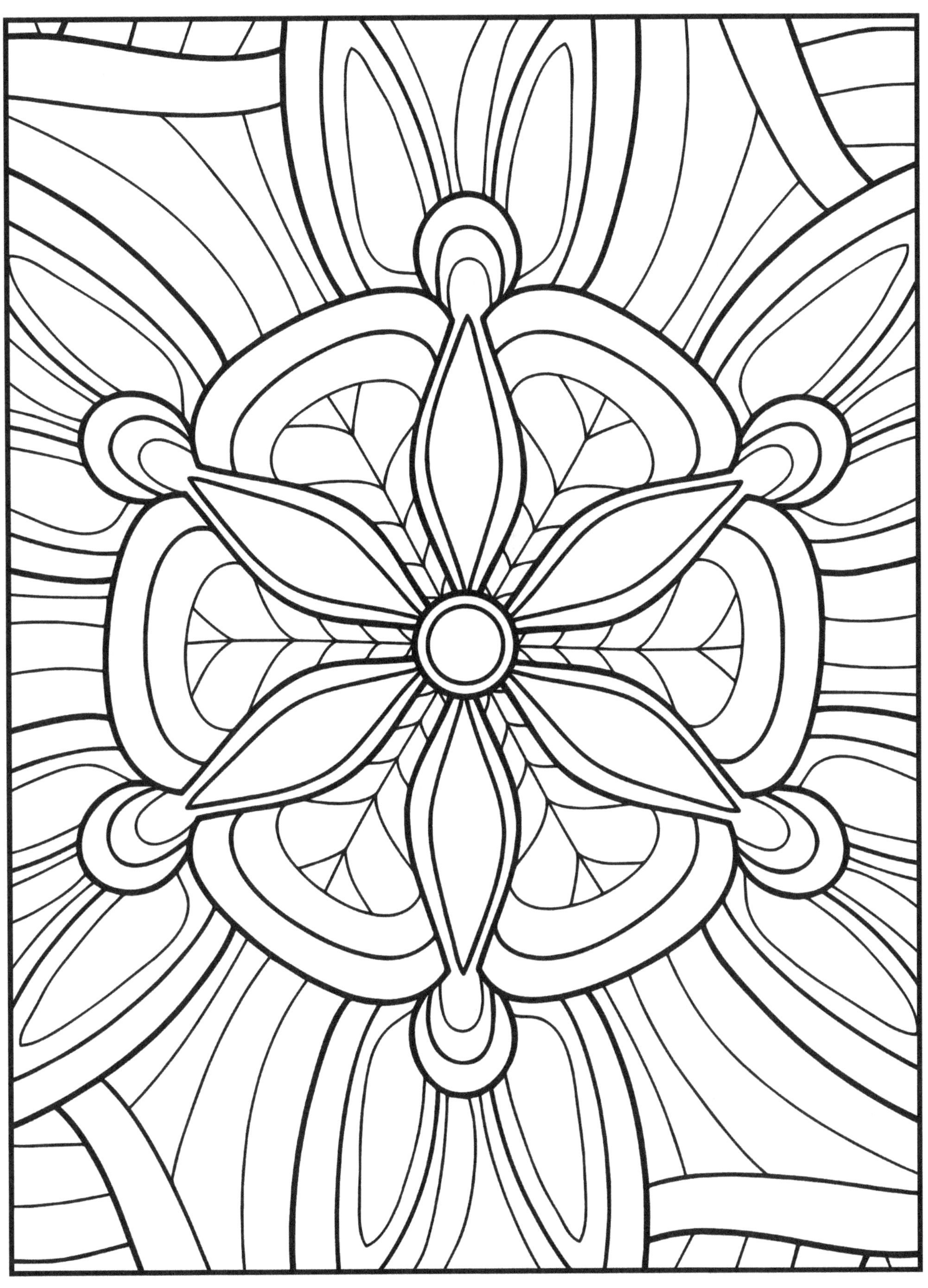

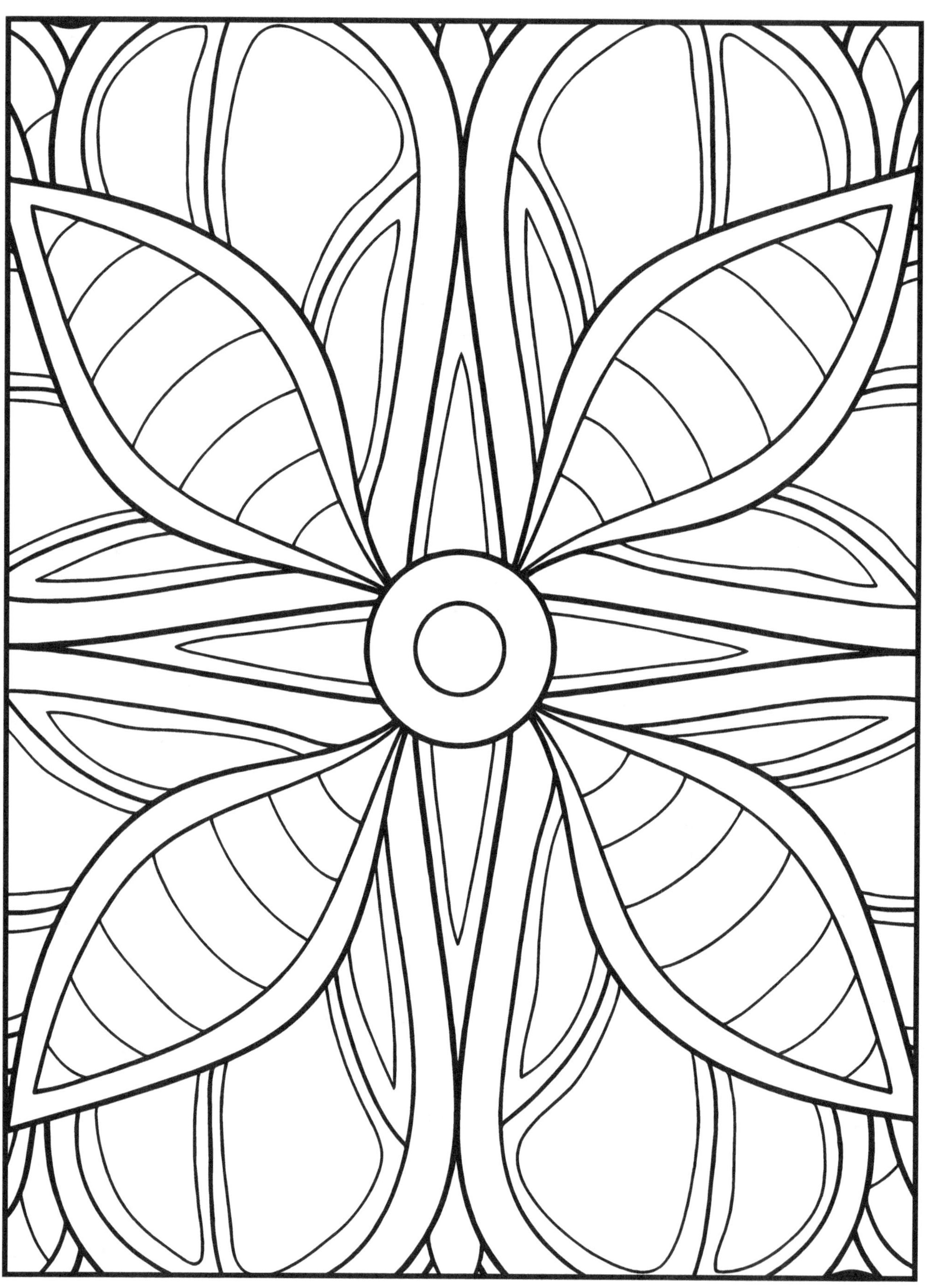

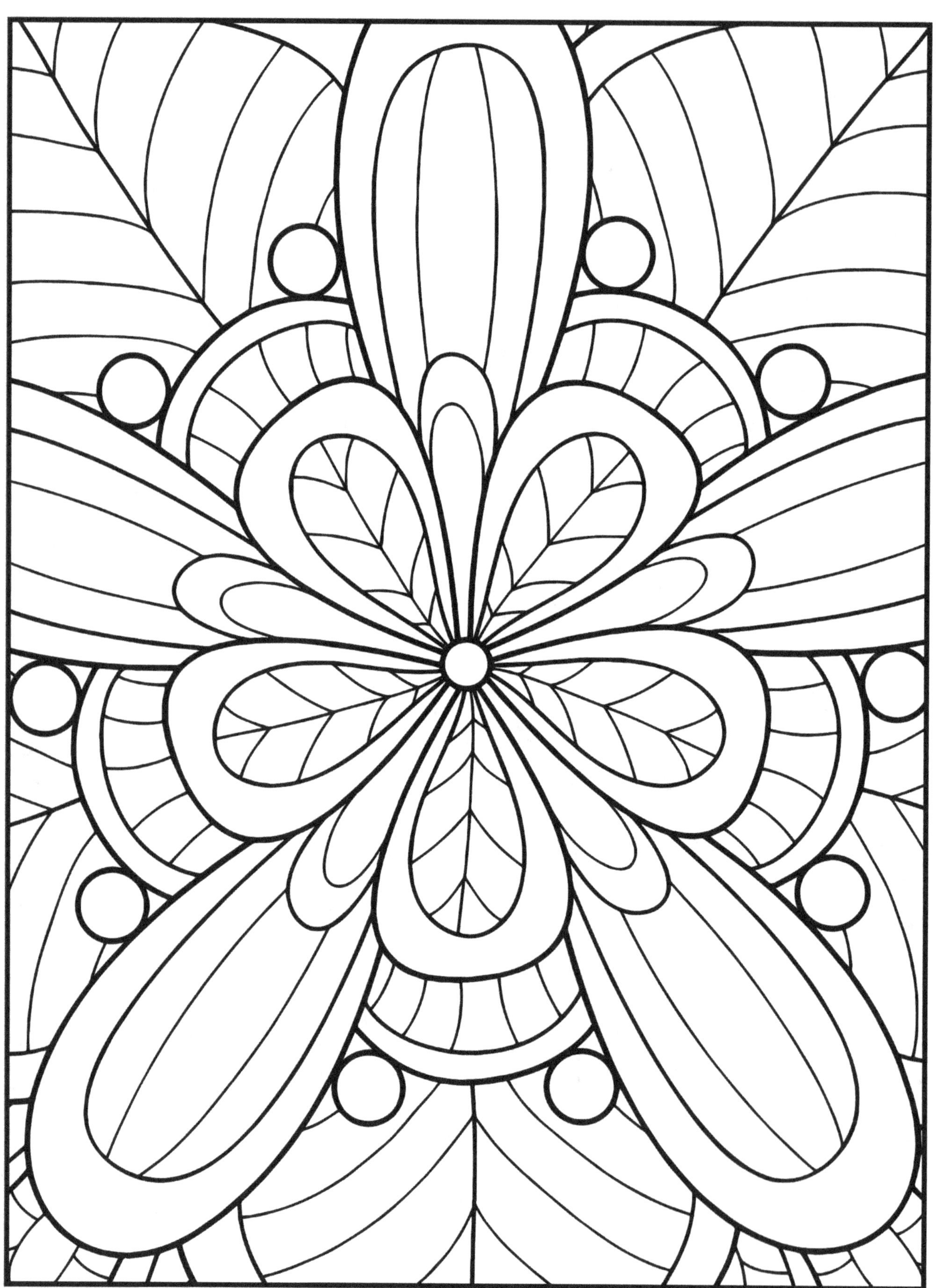

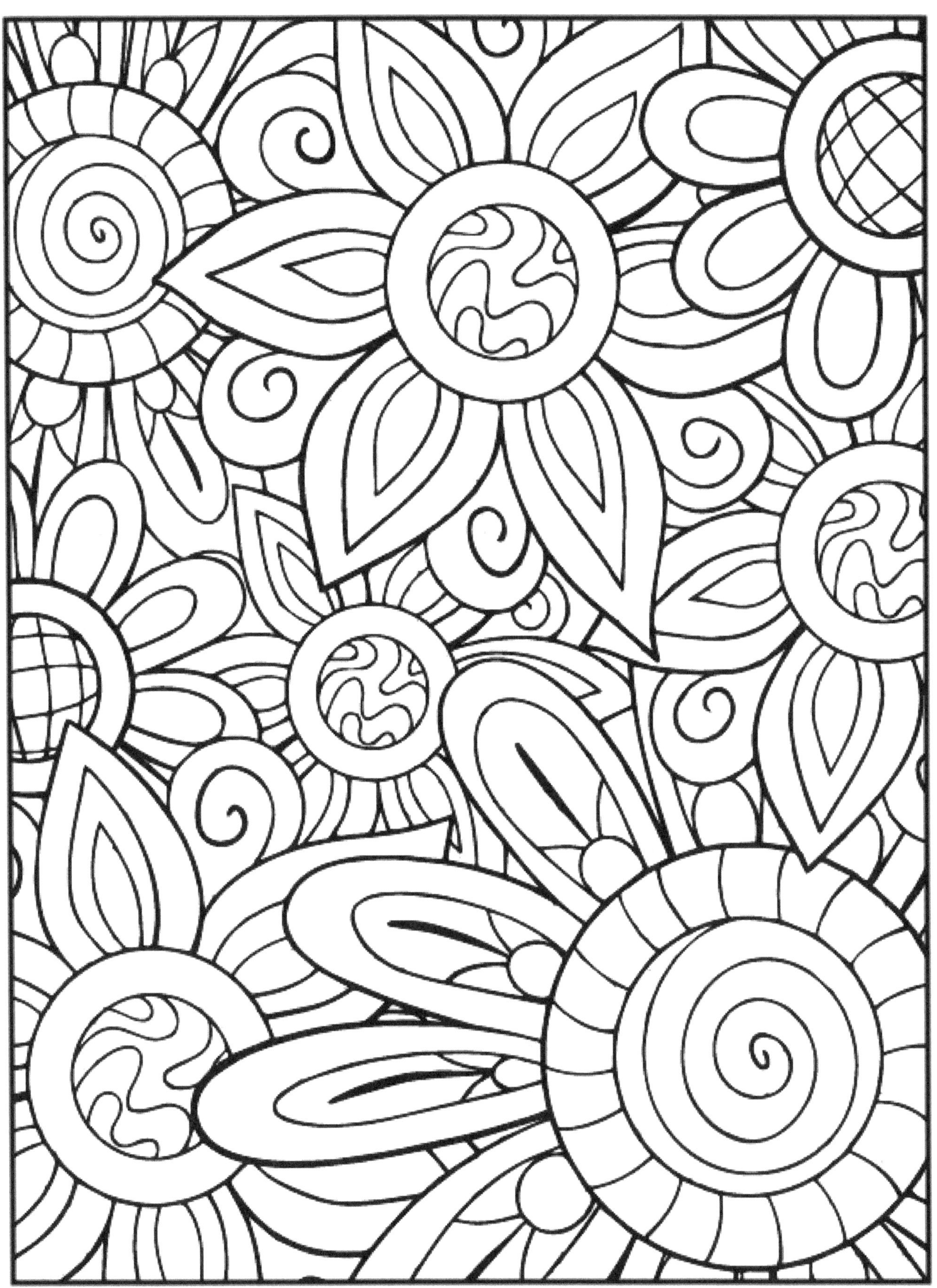

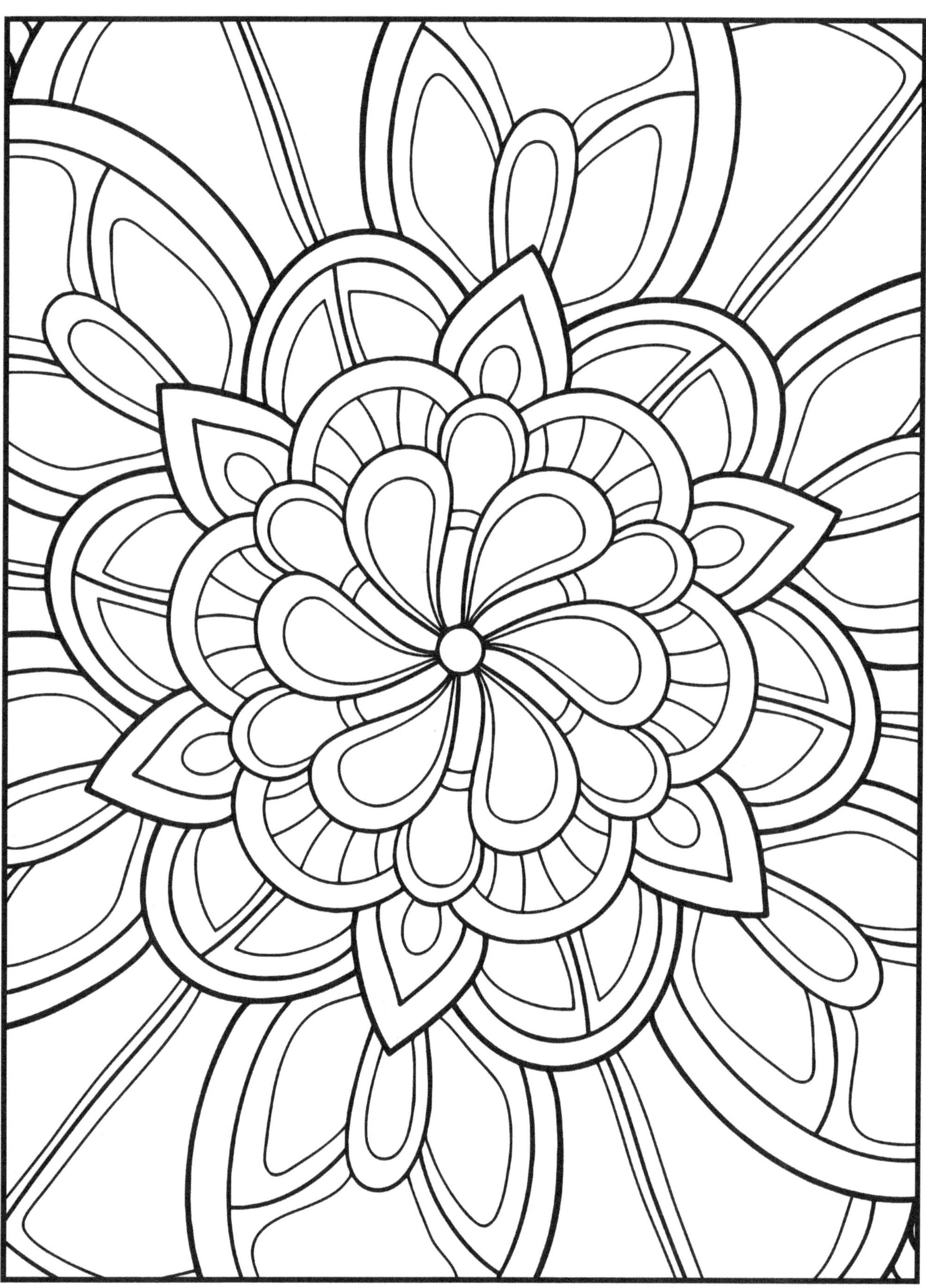

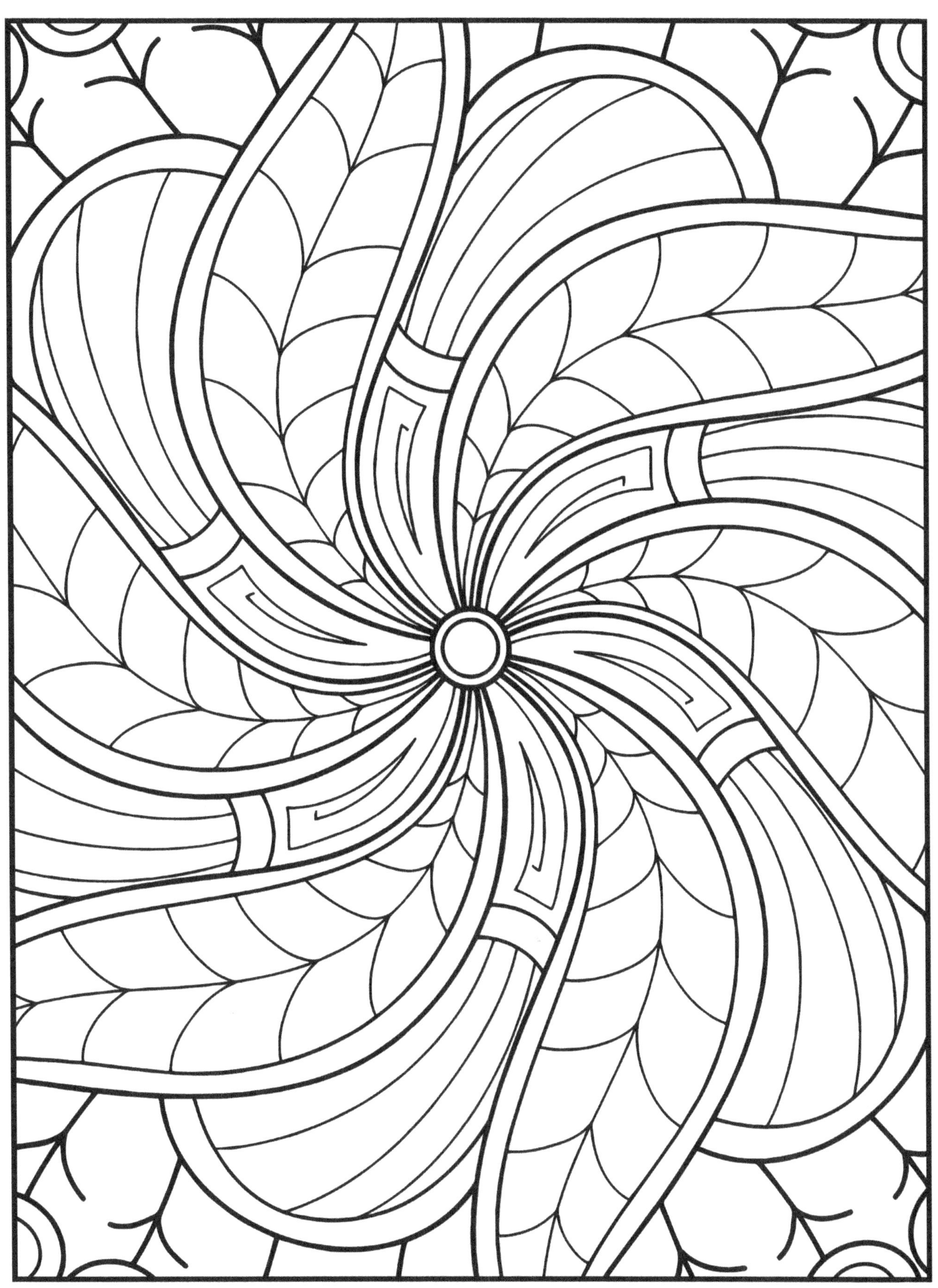

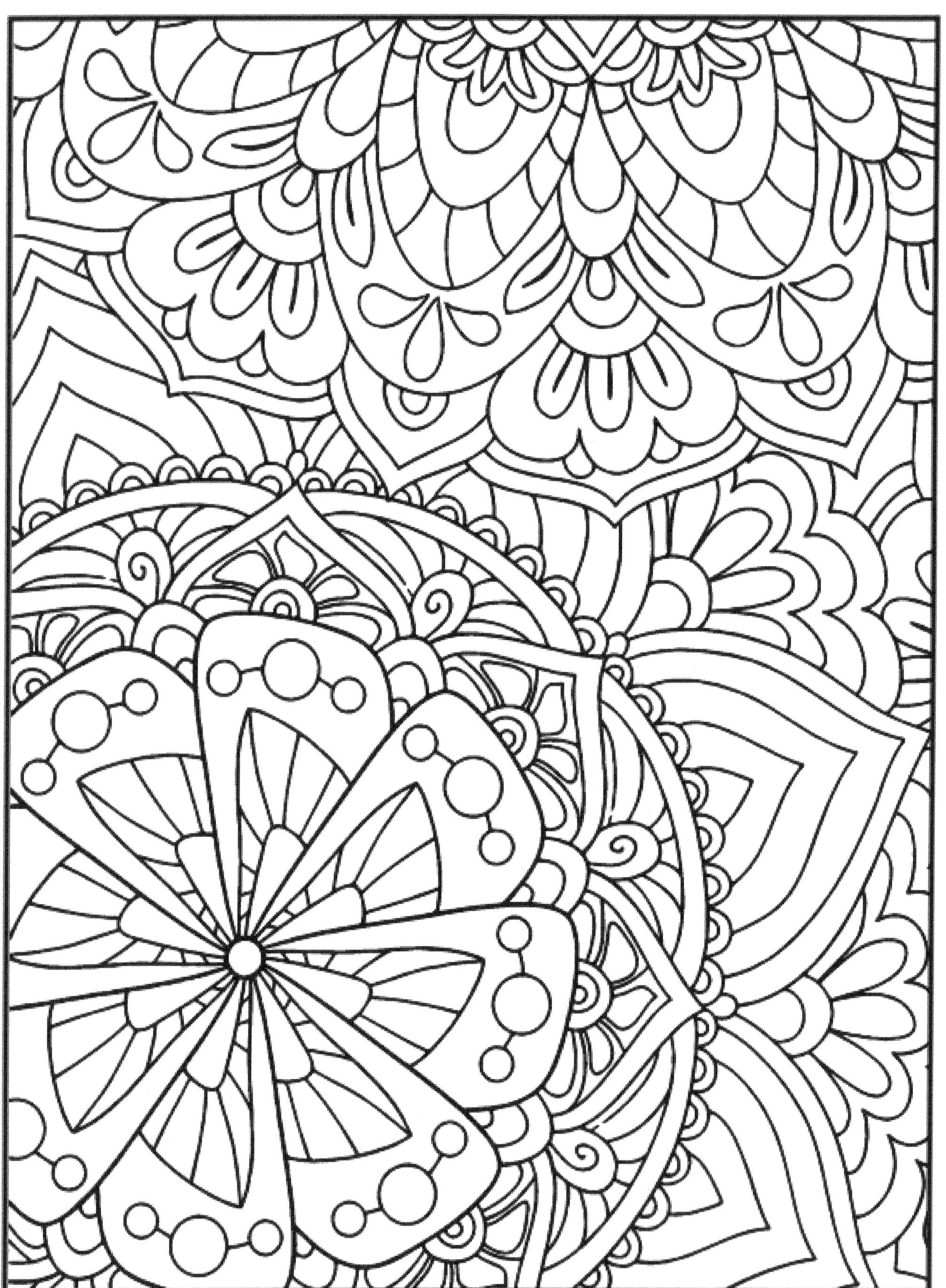

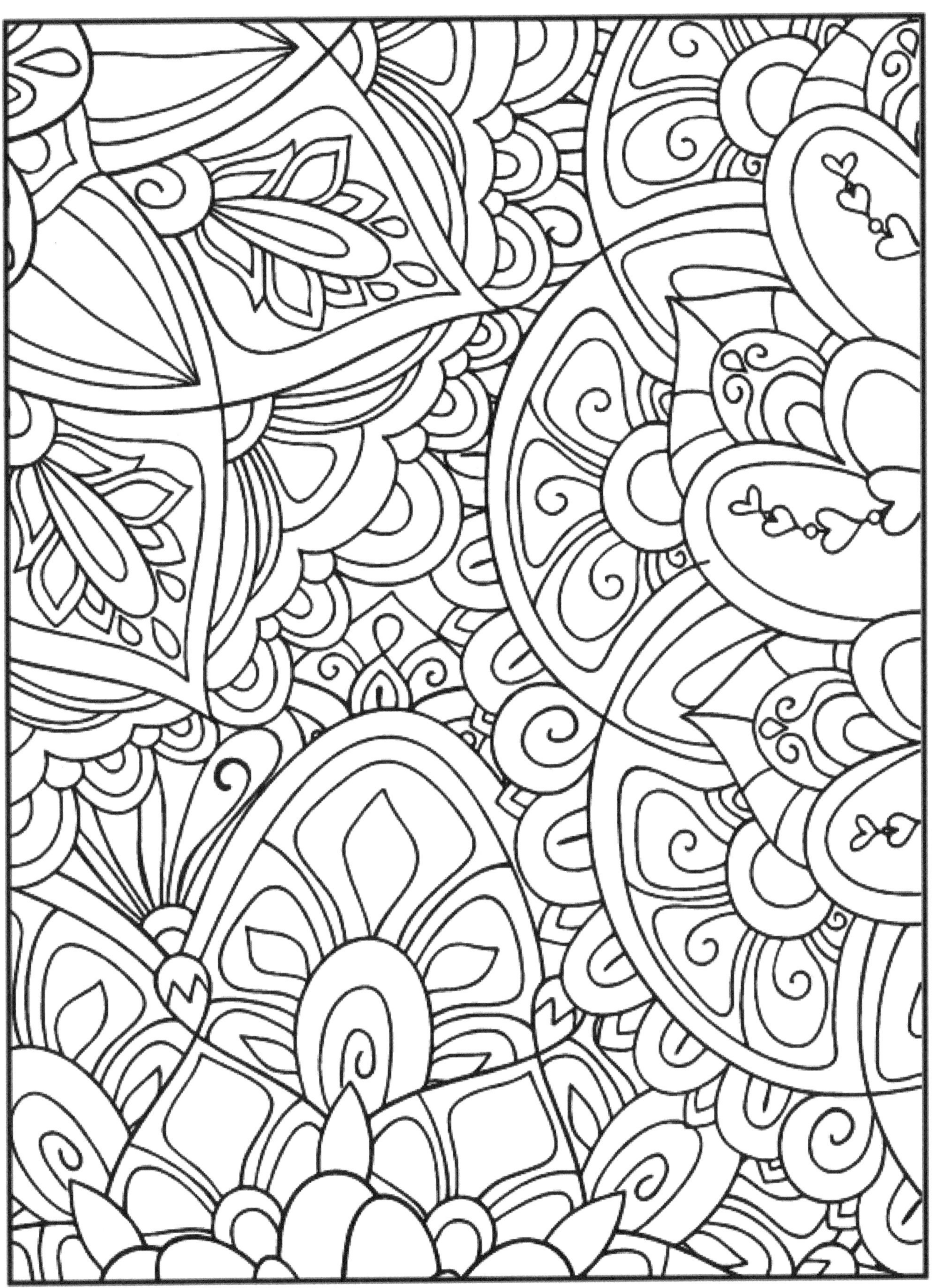

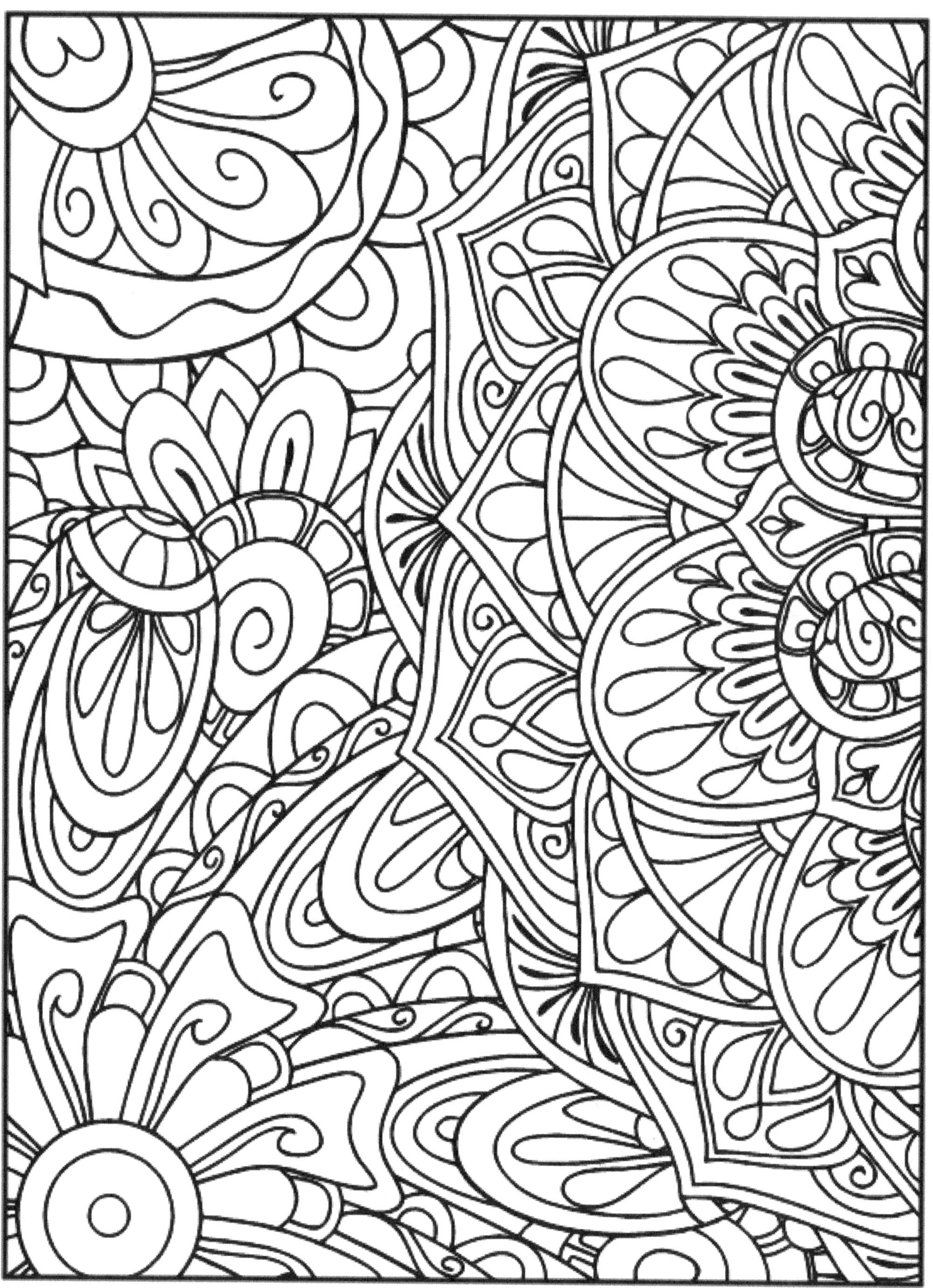

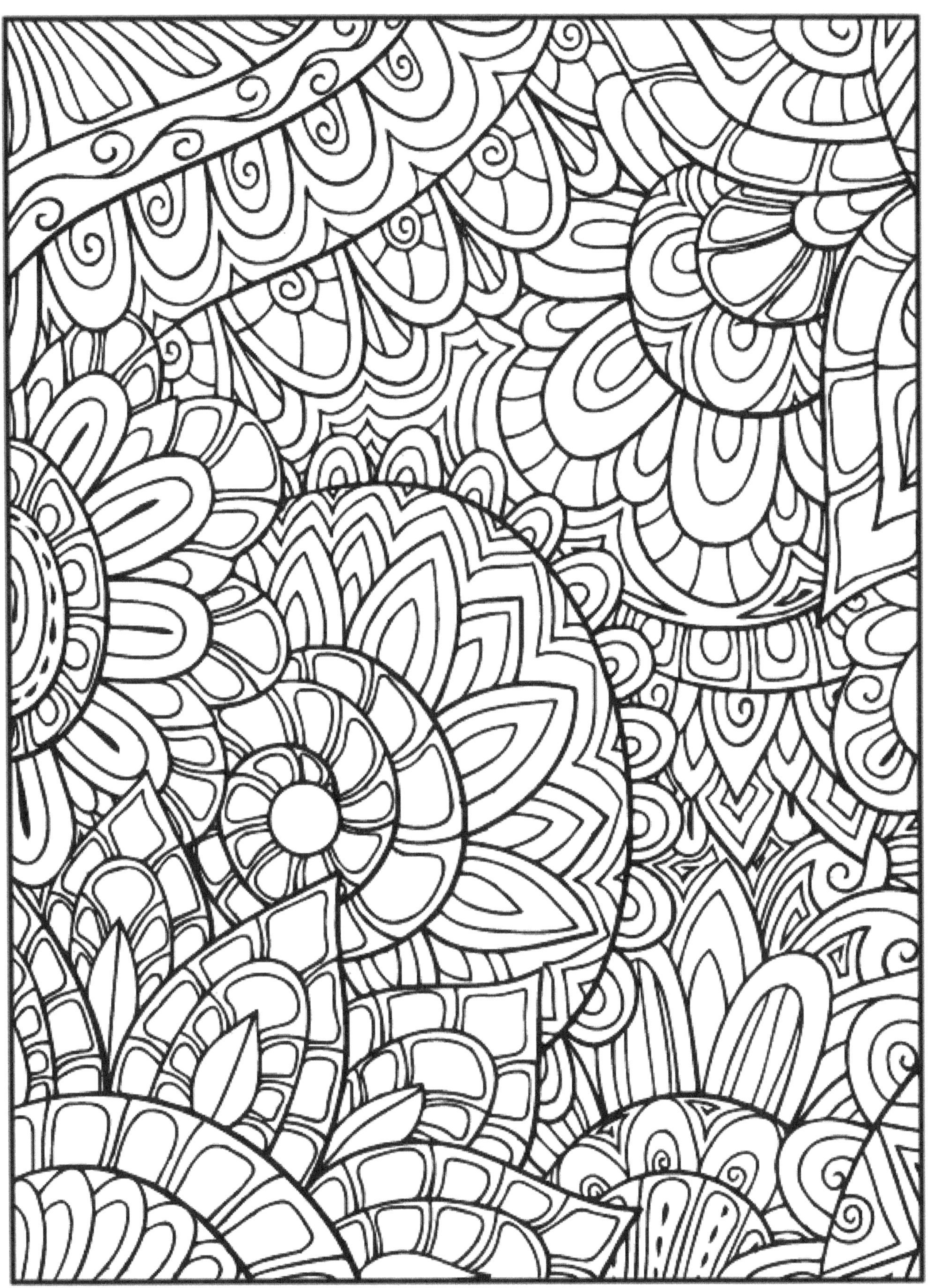

www.ingramcontent.com/pod-product-compliance
Lightning Source LLC
Chambersburg PA
CBHW081603250726
48653CB00009B/3545